Sod Sitting, Get Moving! should be our watchword as we get older. Remember the body is like a machine – full of thousands of moving parts. If you don't keep them well-oiled and moving they will seize up. Be warned!

Angela Rippon, OBE, broadcaster

As I reach the ripe old age of 68, I am only too aware of exercising one's body and mind. I love walking, Pilates and reading. *Sod Sitting, Get Moving!* is the book to make sure that you can make activity fun – and you'll live longer.

Christopher Biggins, national treasure and King of the Jungle

As we get older it's important to keep exercise going if we want to have a healthy life. A half hour walk every day can do us a lot of good. So that it doesn't become a chore it's worth doing something you really enjoy. For me it's swimming, and at the same time you can do lots of exercises which are much more gentle when you try them under the water. Get yourself a dog and get him/her to take you for a good stroll every day. Remember the old saying – use it or lose it – and *Sod Sitting, Get Moving!*

David Hamilton, broadcaster

I have always been a great believer in a healthy lifestyle and have been exercising since I was a young child growing up in Sri Lanka. Now in my sixties I swim every day and train with weights at least three times a week. Exercise is so important to us all and *Sod Sitting, Get Moving!* should be the bible for anyone over fifty. Get moving – it really is fun!

David Wilkie, MBE, Olympic and Commonwealth Games champion

Sod Sitting, Get Moving! is a book for everyone – but particularly for those in later years. As a working GP I see an increasing number of patients in their seventies and beyond. I recommend exercise as the first step to getting better. If we all took the advice in this excellent book we wouldn't need to prescribe quite so many pills.

Dr Dawn Harper, GP, TV presenter and author

Sod Sitting, Get Moving! is a masterclass in motivation. I exercise and train a minimum of four times a week. It gives me a sense of wellbeing and makes me aware of my working body. It really has kept me youthful and I intend to carry on. I urge everyone to *Sod Sitting, Get Moving!* as Diana's book enthuses.

Jacques Azagury, designer

Exercise is normally such a bore, but dancing is wonderful exercise and such fun. Exercise is even better when you move to music, as Diana recommends in this wonderful book. Buy it now and put a spring in your step.

Lionel Blair, entertainer

I've known Diana Moran for years – and in her seventies she still looks in her fifties. If her secret is in this book I thoroughly recommend it. I'm fast realising that the older we get the more we need to stay active!

Matthew Wright, broadcaster

I know seventy is not much of an age nowadays. But when it actually happens to you (me), it's still a bit of a facer. So I agree that Diana's message should be a maxim for us all! And here are my simple exercises for the face: 1. Look up, not down. 2. Look forward, not back. 3. Raise the sides of the mouth. Hold for thirty years. I don't know whether they work, but I'm keeping on with them just in case.

Sir Richard Stilgoe, singer and songwriter

This book is a bible for anyone over sixty. As it recommends, I walk fast every single day for a minimum of half an hour and it has become such a part of my life that I barely notice it. I tend to shop locally so will always walk there and back; if I need to get a bus somewhere I'll walk a couple of stops further than I need to. I feel fitter than I've ever done, my weight has stayed the same for years and I sleep well. It costs nothing and you don't need special equipment. So *Sod Sitting, Get Moving!* – it's worked for me.

Trudie Goodwin, The Bill and Emmerdale actress

At 58 I know the need to keep active – whoever you are. I'm lucky to have maintained my fitness, I don't push the competitive boundaries these days, I just find joy in being active and being able to be active! As Diana recommends in her excellent book, activity can often just be simply walking and having the time and opportunity to commune with nature. Sod Sitting – get active!"

Kriss Akabusi, MBE, athlete and gold medallist

SOD

SITTING, GET MOVING!

GETTING ACTIVE IN YOUR 60s, 70s AND BEYOND

DIANA MORAN AND MUIR GRAY

Illustrated by David Mostyn

Green
Tree

BLOOMSBURY

LONDON · OXFORD · NEW YORK · NEW DELHI · SYDNEY

Green Tree
An imprint of Bloomsbury Publishing Plc

50 Bedford Square
London
WC1B 3DP
UK

1385 Broadway
New York
NY 10018
USA

www.bloomsbury.com

Green Tree is the health, fitness and personal well-being imprint of
Bloomsbury Publishing Plc
BLOOMSBURY and the Diana logo are trademarks of Bloomsbury Publishing Plc

First published in 2017
© Diana Moran and Muir Gray, 2017
Illustrations by David Mostyn

British Library Cataloguing-in-Publication Data
A catalogue record for this book is available from the British Library.

ISBN: Print: 978-1-4729-4376-7
ePDF: 978-1-4729-4378-1
ePub: 978-1-4729-4377-4

4 6 8 10 9 7 5 3

Typeset in FS Me by Deanta Global Publishing Services, Chennai, India
Printed and bound in Great Britain by CPI Group (UK) Ltd. Croydon, CR0 4YY

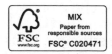

To find out more about our authors and books visit www.bloomsbury.com.
Here you will find extracts, author interviews, details of forthcoming
events and the option to sign up for our newsletters.

CONTENTS

FOREWORD BY AGE UK

There is no magic formula for staying mentally and physically fit and well in later life, but a healthy lifestyle that includes regular exercise, a balanced diet and an active social life are all important factors.

It is also true that it is never too late to start, and that becoming more physically active can actually reverse the decline in areas such as muscle strength and cognitive function.

It's time to challenge the idea that the best thing for older people is to 'sit down and put their feet up'. Of course that's fine sometimes, but sitting less and being active by doing something you enjoy for even 10 minutes will bring big rewards, even if it's a big effort to get started.

This book is co-authored by Age UK's ambassador Diana Moran and Muir Gray, one of the UK's leading doctors on the interaction between ageing, disease, and loss of fitness. It is full of helpful ideas and advice about living well in mind and body as we age and enjoying later life to the full.

Scientists say our genes only make a 25% contribution to the length of life and that factors like lifestyle and nutrition account for the remaining three quarters, so there's lots to be gained from being healthy and active and whatever your age may be – now is a great time to start.

For more information on Age UK, or for details about their Healthy living guide, please visit: www.ageuk.org.uk or phone 0800 169 6565.

SIXTY PLUS? TIME TO GET MOVING

Muir Gray

You are 60 plus – you're at a good time of life – some would say in the prime of life. Surveys have shown that people aged 70 to 74 report the best feelings about life. People in their 60s face more pressures. Many are still supporting their parents, often far away, and still have children dependent on them. They are part of the sandwich generation. People in their 70s rarely have worries about elderly parents, but often still worry about their children and sometimes the chicks return to the nest. Some people, of course, have to cope with the disability or death of a partner, but it is a good time for most people in their 70s.

For people in their 80s life is tougher, with health problems playing a bigger part, but the image of life from 60 onwards being dominated by disease, disability, dependency and dementia is wrong. OK, so you may be a bit slower than you were because of a dodgy hip, you may be a bit more forgetful or you may have a more serious condition, such as arthritis or diabetes, but it is important to remember that people in their 60s, 70s and 80s are a key group in society. For one thing, if they gave up caring for other people the NHS would collapse, tomorrow.

Of course, life could be better; and many people over 60 would benefit from a higher income. Unfortunately, poverty is still too common a problem in old age but that's true for almost everyone, not just people in their 60s, and anyway that's not what this book is about. This book is about giving you the good news, that life can get better without a windfall from the Lottery. Diana Moran and I are both in our 70s, and we've spent our lives studying, preventing and even evangelising about the benefits of exercise and the good it can do for us.

Whatever your age or your income, whether or not you have one or more long-term conditions, and five or ten prescriptions, becoming more active and taking more exercise will:

- Help you feel better

- Reduce your risk of many common health problems, such as heart disease, stroke, depression and, best news of all, dementia

- Make the treatment for any condition or disease more effective, and can sometimes lead to the need for pills disappearing completely

- Improve both your mood and your brain function – how you think and feel

Fantastic, but why isn't exercise available on the NHS, like pills and X-rays? Well, it's not yet, but it is coming because the medical profession is finally waking up to the potential benefits of exercise. Of course, you need to do other things to feel better and stay well, to live longer and aim for a good death as well as a good life, but this book is your guide to exercise – the miracle cure. About half of people aged 60 plus have one or more than one condition, so at your next appointment ask your GP or the hospital doctor you see about whether exercise will help you deal with your particular condition. The answer will almost always be 'yes'. I suggest looking at the NHS Choices website: www.nhs.uk. Type in the name of your condition and, whether it is diabetes or depression,

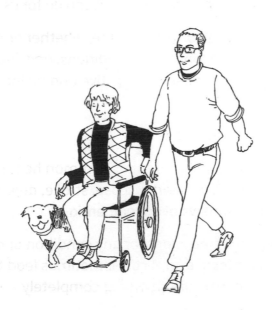

somewhere in that excellent web knowledge service you will find encouragement to be more active.

What's your plan?

The first thing you should do is reflect on where you are in life and where you would prefer to finish up.

One of the myths about older people is that they live in the past. Of course, this is not true. However, the evidence suggests that, with the exception of financial matters, not enough older people think ahead. OK, so if you have children, you quickly work out how to leave as much to the family as you can without incurring the wrath of inheritance tax. But what about planning your future health and well-being, including how you prefer to die, or, even more important, how you hope not to die?

Take a moment to reflect on the following question: How would you prefer to meet your end?

Would you like to:

1. Pop off without warning?

2. Spend the last months, or even years, unable to dress or get to the toilet without help?

3. Stay fit and independent, then have a short final illness?

Why not pause and discuss the options with someone who will be affected by your death? How did you rank the options? The prospect of months or years of immobility and dependence would be at the bottom of everyone's list, and many people like the idea of popping off without warning, preferably on the way home from the perfect holiday on which you had spent the last of your money! However, sudden death leaves many unhappy people behind. There are bereaved family members who never had the chance to tell the person who died how much they loved them and was helped by them, or heard that person say 'I love you' or 'I forgive you'. The best of the three ways of dying is the short final illness, which gives everyone the chance to say their goodbyes.

Towards the end of the 20th century there was growing concern that the recommended strategy of risk reduction, including avoiding physical activity, was just keeping people alive to a miserable advanced old age, condemning those in their 90s to years of disability and dependence. However, recent research points firmly in a completely different direction. Increasing the frequency and intensity of exercise will not only reduce the risk of an early death; it will also:

- Keep you fitter for longer and reduce the time you will be dependent on others

- Help you feel better next month, and every month after that

So, let's get moving more, now. But you know this already don't you? It is obvious, so why are you now taking less exercise than you did when you were 20, or less exercise

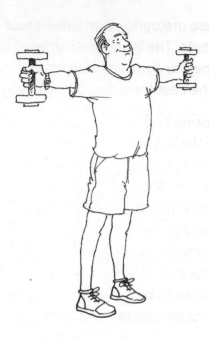

than you know, or think, will transform your health?
Here are the most common reasons people give for not
exercising enough, and our solutions to the problem.

Your good reason: *I don't have the time*
Our response: We understand that but you owe it to
yourself to manage your time better so as to give a little
bit more to yourself. Just ten minutes every morning
will give you enough time for our Triple S, Strength Skill
and Suppleness programme. And ten more minutes
focused on brisk walking, once, or better still, twice, or
(best) three times a day for the fourth s – stamina.

Your good reason: *I can't afford it*
Our response: Although we recommend weights
and resistance bands or classes in techniques such

as Pilates, these are optional extras – good ideas for birthday presents. The exercises can be done without spending money, or by using a big bag of flour or sugar as a weight (the best thing to do with a bag of sugar!).

Your good reason: *I have not enjoyed exercise in the past*
Our response: We will help you understand the benefits. You are not doing physical activity because it is fun (although it can be). Think of it as training for the decades to come. Athletes train for the Olympics; you are in training for your eighties and that will be a big event. We also recommend you do it with a buddy or two. Even when doing your daily dozen on your own at home, find some other friends to do it at the same time. They will feel the same as you; be a bit supportive and a bit competitive.

Your good reason: *I am too busy helping other people*
Our response: We know how much people in our age group do for grandchildren, children, parents, partners, neighbours and the community, but they need you to look after yourself too. In addition, it will help your children and grandchildren considerably if you are still active and independent in your eighties, so getting fitter is part of looking after those you love and care for.

Healthcare is what people do for themselves, and one of the best types of healthcare is to get moving!

Now, the first step is not to get up out of your chair and go for a walk, although it is good to stand and stretch if you have been sitting down for 15 minutes or more. The first step is to understand what is going on inside your body

as the years pass. In times past, growing older was seen
and often portrayed in pictures as a time of increasing
inactivity, of sitting dozing by the fireside. But what we
now know now has led to the development of a new
approach based on new facts about ageing and activity.

The new facts of life – the birds and the bees – for people over 60

The new facts of life are:

- First, that physical activity is more important for
  people in their 60s, 70s, 80s, 90s and beyond than
  it is for people in their 20s and 30s

- Second, that it is at least as important to try to
  increase fitness after the onset of disease as it
  is to try to prevent disease through increased
  activity

This is nothing short of a revolution in how we think
about growing older, and that revolution has to be led
by older people. The most important fact to understand
is that ageing is not the cause of all the problems that
are more common in older adults. Until the age of 90
the biological process of ageing has little effect on your
ability to look after yourself, engage with other people or
get about independently. If you reach the age of 90 and
are affected only by ageing you will be independent and
active, and even in work, like Her Majesty The Queen or
David Attenborough, for example. Some decline in ability
is inevitable but the rate at which our abilities decline

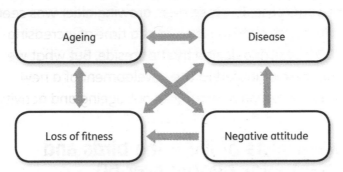

How a negative attitude affects fitness

is influenced not only by ageing but also by three other processes which do cause problems – disease, loss of fitness and a negative attitude to life – and all three are interrelated.

The most important of these processes is what you believe and your attitude to life.

Strengthening and keeping your positive attitude

A pessimistic attitude and outlook on life is influenced by the negative, and incorrect, portrayal of 'old age' as a period of inevitable and irreversible decline by most media. A pessimistic attitude does accelerate the rate of the decline however, partly because people who adopt this attitude make no attempt to get fitter, let alone keep fit, nor do they try to reduce the risk of disease.

Some people, unfortunately including some doctors, say 'It's your age' or, even worse, 'what else do you expect at your age?' These statements are examples of ageism, and although we have heard less about ageism than racism or sexism, it is moving up the agenda. Ageism is a prejudice and a prejudice comes from the term 'prejudging', namely judging someone on the basis of one characteristic before you know what they're really like.

The first point to make is that people who are 60 or 70, or any age for that matter, differ from one another in many ways, so all generalisations have to be taken with a very big pinch of salt. The second point is that such statements are based on the false belief that all problems are due to the ageing process. This belief is widespread and influences many people, including many older people.

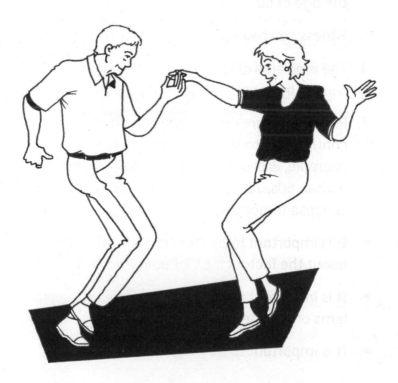

So, always remember that *you* are *you*; never mind whatever other people think. You need to believe in yourself and in these magnificent seven facts:

1. Ageing by itself is not a major cause of disability itself until the 90s

2. Many of the problems that we have assumed are due to ageing are due to loss of fitness

3. Many of the problems that we have assumed are due to ageing are due to preventable disease

4. The risk of disease can still be reduced after the age of 60

5. Fitness can be regained after the age of 60

6. The problems of too many older people are caused by deprivation and poverty, not ageing

7. People who are over 60 make a positive contribution to society in many ways; for example, without the contribution of people in their 60s, 70s, 80s and older the NHS would collapse tomorrow

- It is important to be clear in your own mind about the factors that influence your abilities

- It is important not to feel guilty about the problems of younger people

- It is important to be positive and optimistic.

The fitness gap and how to close it

'What has fitness got to do with me?' I hear you say. Well, there are two answers to that. First, physical activity is a good antidote to depression and it increases the probability that you will feel well in the short term (as well as making your muscles and heart work better). However, getting more active is also an insurance programme for the long term. This insures you against the risk of becoming incontinent, dependent on other people, and becoming a burden to your nearest and dearest – possibly the biggest fear of all!

The good news is that whatever your age you can close the fitness gap between the best possible rate of decline, which only a few very fit people follow, and the actual rate of decline.

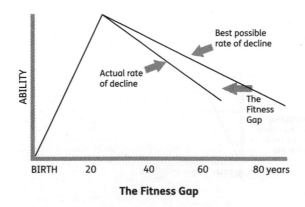

The Fitness Gap

There has been little or no research into fitness for centenarians, but the anecdotal evidence is persuasive. Many of those who have made it to three figures are certain that they have reached the milestone by keeping themselves active. There are, however, some studies of people in their 90s and very many studies of people in their 80s, 70s and 60s, all of which have the same very encouraging message – whatever your age, you can get fitter and improve your level of ability, as shown in the figure below.

The scientific evidence about the benefits of training is very strong, and has been for decades. Twenty years ago Professor Roy J. Shephard published his classic book *Ageing, Physical Activity and Health*. His message is clear and unequivocal – by becoming more active 'biological age is effectively reduced by as much as 10 to 20 years.'

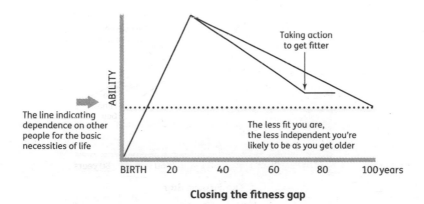

Closing the fitness gap

There are four aspects to fitness, all of which can be improved:

1. Stamina: how long you can keep going

2. Skill: how well you can co-ordinate your actions, for example when recovering from a stumble

3. Suppleness: the opposite of stiffness

4. Strength: what your muscles can do (and power: how quickly they can do it)

Getting fitter and keeping fit are high priorities and the new message from research is that getting fitter may be even more important for people with one or more than one disease or condition than it is for people who have managed to avoid developing any condition.

Getting fitter is both a means of prevention and a type of treatment.

Disease: reducing the risk and coping with it

Disease occurs more often in older age groups, and although some of these diseases are related to the ageing process, most of them are due to a different cause: having lived for a long time. This is not the same thing.

The more years you live with a bad diet or in an unhealthy environment the greater the likelihood that you will develop a disease. But this is not a result of ageing.

The wake-up call for many people is the diagnosis of high blood pressure or Type 2 diabetes or any of the other modern epidemics. This is the kick in the pants that they need. Sixty per cent of people aged 60 have a condition such as this, as do more than 70 per cent of people aged 70 and above. And, as the decades go by, the percentage of people having *more* than one condition increases. But what do we mean by 'conditions' and how do they relate to disease?

Once upon a time diseases were pretty clear-cut. You either had tuberculosis or a broken leg or you didn't. However, medicine has changed over the years as the population has aged. Now we use the word 'condition' to mean a state in which your health is impaired or you are at risk of some serious complication, even though you didn't know you had it until a doctor or nurse told you.

High blood pressure is an example of a condition; so too is Type 2 diabetes. By this we mean that there is not a

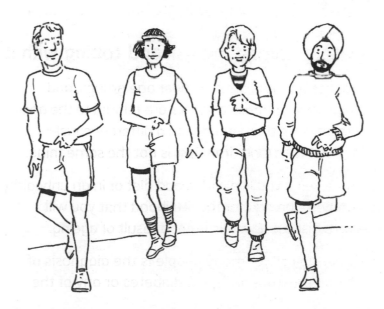

sharp cut-off point between people with the condition and people without it. Identifying high blood pressure as a problem comes through measuring your blood pressure. But doctors and nurses have arbitrary limits about the level of blood pressure. So, when they say, 'You have got high blood pressure, I'm afraid,' what they should really say is, 'Your level of blood pressure is such that there is an increased risk of stroke and dementia. I recommend you consider taking medication to reduce it. Although I have to warn you that the medication itself has side effects. And although you have not noticed this increase in your blood pressure, you may well notice the effects of taking the medicine that I could prescribe to bring it down.'

An even better response from the doctor might be: 'Your blood pressure is not dangerously high, so before I offer you drug treatment, I would like to suggest you start a fitness programme. Physical activity combined with associated weight loss might bring your blood pressure down and avoid the need for drug treatment.'

This is, of course, quite a long rigmarole but it is something that doctors are increasingly saying to people. Many conditions of modern life are caused by the environment. This environment leads to inactivity, which in turn leads to the steady increase in weight that so many people experience from the age of 20 onwards.

While it is important to understand the distinction between a condition and a disease, there are, of course, diseases that are still quite distinct and different – rheumatoid arthritis, for example, or parkinson's. But the simple fact is that we need to be thinking about fitness for both conditions and diseases. Even if these diseases reduce your ability to move and make it more difficult to take exercise, the scientific evidence is now clear that increasing physical activity is essential, and never more so than after the onset of a condition or disease. Sometimes, exercise is at least as important as the medical treatment itself.

Some diseases, such as arthritis, do reduce your ability to exercise, as shown in the figure below. But we also find that people lose fitness more quickly after the onset of their condition or disease than before it.

After all the good news, it is still the case that too many people are simply given pills when a condition or a disease is diagnosed. Not enough are given pills plus advice on exercise. The medical profession is waking up to this and recently the Academy of Medical Royal Colleges published a major report called 'Exercise – the Miracle Cure'. Yet, despite this, the focus is still on pills and operations in too many consultations, at too many health centres and too many hospital clinics.

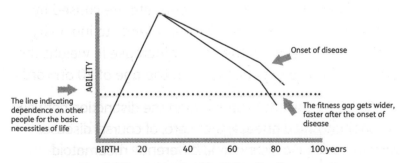

How the fitness gap gets wider faster after disease occurs

On top of this, well-intentioned relatives can add to the problem through their efforts to help. 'Don't you worry about the shopping, dear, I'll do that for you. You don't want to walk to the shops when it might rain.' The new facts of life are that walking to the shops, as briskly as you can, is even more important if you have a long-term condition than if you don't.

If you are living with a long-term health condition and are looking to use exercise as therapy, there's lots of great advice on the big common problems online from the following organisations:

Diabetes UK
Asthma UK
The British Heart Foundation
The Stroke Association
Arthritis Research UK
Parkinson's UK
Macmillan Cancer Support
The Alzheimer's Society
The Lung Foundation
Rethink Mental Illness
MIND
The MS Society

UKActive, the new charity promoting activity, has identified people who are ageing as a priority group and all the key professional groups like the British Geriatrics Society and the Chartered Society of Physiotherapists are now promoting physical activity among older people with health problems. In addition, The Centre for Ageing Better has identified inactivity as a priority and AgeUK does wonderful work. It stimulates many people through their local programmes called Inspire & Include and Get Going Together.

Get moving to better health and slower ageing

So a new approach is needed. Vast sums of money are being spent on the search for the elixir of life, a drug that would slow the ageing process. As yet, there is no such thing. But there is a fascinating new idea emerging from research, namely that by becoming more active we can reduce a biological change that seems to be one of the main causes of what we call the ageing process – inflammation.

We all know about acute inflammation: the swollen, red tenderness round an infected cut. The inflammation of tissue; a characteristic of ageing, has been assumed to be due to the normal ageing process, about which

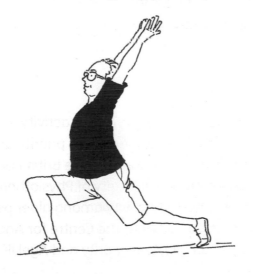

nothing could be done. However, recent studies show that inflammation of key tissues, blood vessels and the brain, for example, can be prevented – and the main means of prevention is, you guessed it, activity.

To understand why getting moving can prevent ageing we need to look at the stress reaction. This is sometimes called the 'fight or flight' reaction. When we were evolving as human beings, life was full of sudden dangers. Our ancestors would always need to be ready to react to an encounter with a sabre-toothed tiger or a hostile neighbouring tribe, for example. The stress reaction then was very helpful, helping you to either take flight and run away quickly, or fight.

Nowadays, such threats are uncommon, but we still have stress in our lives, though today it is often experienced in a situation in which you cannot fight or take flight. And we now know that if you experience stress when you are physically inactive the result is an inflammatory reaction. If, for example, there is a family quarrel or a complaint from a neighbour, and you have to cope with the stress while sitting and inactive, the result is inflammation.

Stress + inactivity = inflammation

The antidote to ageing

The ageing process cannot, as yet, be slowed down. But by focusing on the three other aspects of growing older – loss of fitness, disease and attitude – you can stay young and even feel younger.

Common to all three of these processes is the need to increase activity.

What's going on inside you

'This baby could live to be 142 years old' was the startling caption for a photo of a baby on the cover of *Time* magazine at the end of February 2015. It was a special edition based on 'Dispatches from the Frontiers of Longevity' which contained 'new data on how to live a longer, happier life'.

Perhaps the most important fact is that ageing is not the cause of all the problems that are more common in older adults. There is no doubt that ageing exists as a normal biological process. It starts in the early 20s – as our phase of growth and development comes to an end. The general effect reduces our ability to cope with challenges, such as infection and loss of balance, as well as the biggest challenge of the 21st century – inactivity.

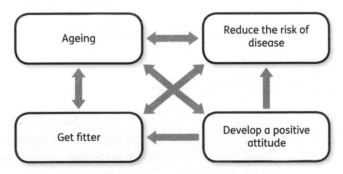

How a positive attitude affects fitness

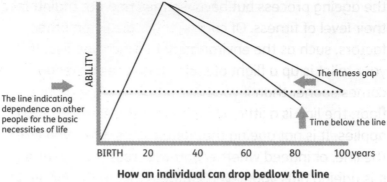

**How an individual can drop bedlow the line
solely owing to loss of fitness**

Keeping above the line

During their phase of development our children are dependent on us. Now, that phase of dependence seems, to many parents at least, to be increasing, as the rising cost of housing forces an increasing proportion of young people to stay in the family nest for longer. However, unlike small children, at least our grown up children are able to dress themselves, clean their teeth, get to the toilet in time and feed themselves (even if they can't yet do their laundry!). They are above the line – the dreaded line that marks our level of ability. When we fall below the line we then become increasingly and depressingly dependent on other people.

The importance of fitness is that it can determine when you drop below the line or whether or not you drop below it at all, as shown in the figure above. This poor person dropped below the line at which they could reach the toilet in time at the age of 78. This wasn't because of the ageing process but because they had not maintained their level of fitness. Of course, there are often other factors, such as the environment in which you live. If your toilet is up a flight of stairs, then the challenge comes sooner than if you have a toilet on the ground floor; the line is a little bit higher but the same principle applies. It is not ageing that determines when you cross the line, or indeed whether you will cross the line at all, it is ageing plus your level of fitness. But never forget, the good news is that your level of fitness, and therefore your level of ability, can be improved at any age.

Caring through activity

Millions of people over 60 care for others who are severely affected by disease and disability. In addition, there are many people in care homes because they have been unable to continue coping on their own.

The word 'care' is an important one. Obviously one aspect of the term is something we would all welcome, namely compassion and sympathy. However, caring for someone all too often means doing things for someone, usually with the best of intentions, in order to help them, but often because it is quicker to do so. If you care for someone you should help them to become more active and more independent, and there are a number of ways in which this can be done. Diana Moran has compiled a detailed range of exercises that will be perfect for your needs whatever they are. Read on.

INTRODUCTION

Diana Moran

So, now we know why activity is important, I say, 'Sod sitting – get moving!', right away.

As Muir says in his introduction, being fit is a necessity, not just an option. Your individual level of fitness will depend on your personal lifestyle, interests and the commitment you have to looking after your health. Fitness is all about being able to do the things *you* want when *you* want to. We all need to do what we can to help ourselves maintain physical independence, and one significant but simple way is by including more activity in our everyday lives. The earlier you develop good habits, the more benefit you'll feel as the years roll past.

So make the opportunity to be more active, and take it, anytime, anywhere and in any way.

Try to take more regular moderate exercise, and persuade your friends or family to join you. Start with simple things, like taking the dog for a walk or using the stairs instead of the lifts. Or try walking to work or the shops or to school instead of taking the car. Then you can look forward to enjoying many more years of ACTIVE life. The trick is to do an activity that gives you pleasure. You will then discover that being active actually boosts your energy levels. When we exercise, the body releases chemicals called endorphins which give us a 'feel-good' factor

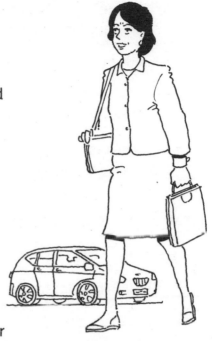

as the circulation gets going, improving our heart and lung efficiency. Exercise and being active makes your complexion glow and your mind more alert. As we've seen, being inactive is a major risk as we get older. Both Muir and I say – 'down with sofas and up with stairs'. Walking is our prescription for good health. Do it with others and help others do it.

Brisk walking

- Lessens the risk of heart disease

- Encourages more oxygen into your lungs

- Improves your cardio-vascular system

- Is 'weight bearing' (body weight is supported by spine, legs and feet)

- Builds healthy bones

- Builds strong leg muscles – vital for physical independence.

- Can be both sociable and beneficial – especially if you have a partner to walk with

How can fitness improve your health?

Physical fitness has five components:

1. Cardio-vascular fitness

2. Muscular strength

3. Muscular endurance

4. Flexibility

5. Motor fitness

Cardio-vascular fitness provides us with stamina. Good stamina enables you to sustain free bodily movement for the length of time you need it without leaving you feeling puffed, exhausted or faint. To achieve good stamina, you must aim to do enough regular activity in order to boost the efficiency of your heart and lungs, and improve your circulation and digestion.

Work on your cardio-vascular fitness by doing aerobic exercises (aerobic exercises simply mean exercising with air). Examples of these types of exercises are:

- Exercises to music (such as line dancing or ballroom dancing)

- Jogging

- Brisk walking

Whichever aerobic exercise or activity you choose, you need to sustain it for a length of time in order to gain benefit. Thirty minutes is an ideal time, but do take age and ability into account. All aerobic activities will make your heart (which itself is a muscle) pump just that little bit harder, and this has the effect of making your lungs work more efficiently, utilising the oxygen you breathe

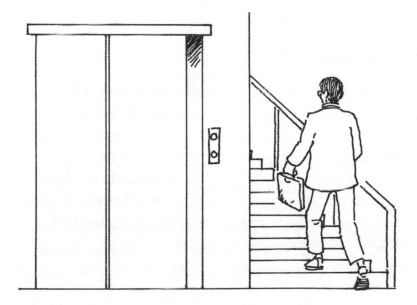

in and improving your circulation. It's important to breathe deeply in order to encourage greater oxygen intake and lung elasticity. Aerobic exercises make you feel warm and puff a bit, but you should still be able to talk while you're doing them!

The second component of physical fitness is **muscular strength**. This is the ability of a muscle to exert maximum force to overcome a resistance. This simply means being able to do things like twisting the stubborn top off a jar of marmalade, or being able to pick up a particularly heavy object. Your body needs strong muscles in order to maintain good posture and improve your shape. As the years advance, it's paramount to keep leg muscles strong. I'd suggest concentrating on strengthening the front thigh muscles (quadriceps) to maintain your physical mobility. Simple regular brisk walking involves the rhythmic movement of both muscles and joints, and will stop the muscles atrophying.

To be physically fit you also need **muscular endurance**. This is the ability of a muscle (or group of muscles) to exert force, in order to overcome a resistance, for an extended period of time. In other words, you need strong muscles to make light work of everyday chores. Those occasions when you have to push yourself just that little bit harder, or exert a little more strength for longer periods than you want, in order to achieve. How many times have I wanted to drop my heavy shopping bags in the supermarket car park just because I have stupidly forgotten where I parked the car? Situations like this call for muscular endurance, and one has to keep on walking and looking. What a relief to finally find the car and be able to put the bags down. If you have well-toned, strong muscles, you reduce the risk of tearing ligaments or damaging yourself when pushed to the limits or if you have a fall.

The next component of physical fitness is **flexibility**. Being flexible enables you to put your muscles and joints through their full range of movements with ease. We take this flexibility or suppleness for granted when we are young, but you need to work at it as you get older. It's a great feeling to be able to use your body efficiently to bend down to do up your shoelaces, to stretch up to high shelves and to use your body to its full potential.

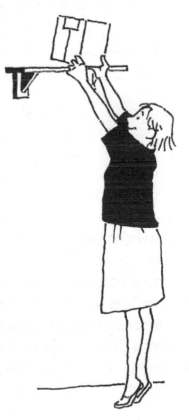

Stretching exercises should be performed before and after an exercise session or physical activity, such as gardening, jogging or playing tennis, in order to prevent injury. When you finish being active your muscles are warm, so it's safe to stretch them out just that little bit more, in order to increase your flexibility and suppleness. Do it at the end of a brisk walk – and surprise yourself by finding you are suppler and able to reach parts you couldn't reach before.

Finally, there's **motor fitness**, which governs your skill and ability to control movements, balance, speed, co-ordination and agility. It gives you the capacity to react quickly, and the confidence to move about without fear of falling over. With skill and the natural co-ordination of mind and body working together you can make your movements graceful, effective and efficient.

If you work hard on all five components of your physical fitness, there is a good chance of maintaining your physical independence long into later life. The benefits to your general health and well-being are enormous and will give you the opportunity to live a full life. In order to maintain your physical fitness, make exercise a natural part of every day. Try to be generally more active: walk more, climb stairs, cycle, dance, swim and garden. Moderate exercise CAN help enhance and maintain your quality of life. But there are no quick fixes for a healthy lifestyle, just two simple rules: be more active and eat sensibly.

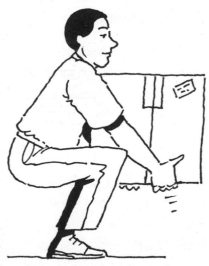

1

GETTING OLDER: YOUR CHOICES

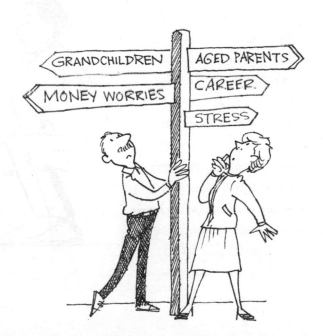

As the years go by, your circumstances will inevitably change: you may move to a smaller house or away from your friends; you may be diagnosed with a condition or a disease; you may just become a little slower and a bit more fragile. In these situations, you have two choices: sink or swim. For example, many people find themselves living alone, sometimes through choice, but more often through divorce or the death of their partner. This situation can lead to loneliness, depression and isolation. It takes a great deal of self-motivation to get out of the spiral of depression. Getting out and talking to people can help to lift depression, while social interaction and the ability to share problems can raise the spirits for all of us. Whatever your situation, it is important to decide to be a 'positive ager' – to relish your individualism, be open-minded and eager to embrace all the opportunities that life still has to offer. Some retired people get bored and fatigued after years of hard work and are lost as to how to spend their time. Waking up in the morning they see long

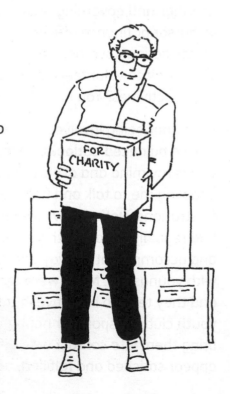

days stretching before them with nothing planned, but it doesn't have to be that way.

Engaging in social and productive activities, like volunteering in the community, can help maintain well-being. Think what interests, skills or knowledge you have to offer, and look for places to volunteer. You might like to read with children at your local primary school, get involved in local politics, or your parish or local council, volunteer at a food bank or in a charity shop on the high street, get more involved in your church, synagogue or mosque activities – there are so many good ways to use your time. If you have financial skills, there are charities and governing bodies crying out for your help as bursar or finance officer. Local schools are also keen on attracting governors, and maybe now is the time to get back into volunteering at guiding, scouting or other youth activities? You have the time now!

I find that being involved with younger people helps me have a balanced outlook on life, and listening to them opens my mind and avoids me getting set in my ways, enabling me to talk and help sort out their problems and frustrations. Notice how older men and women who've had regular contact with young people have a relaxed and accommodating way about them when dealing with youngsters. Many were teachers or organisers, and they tend to be active in their social lives, running youth clubs or sports or hobby-orientated events that bring them into contact with different generations. They appear satisfied and fulfilled, not becoming bigoted and disillusioned with today's youth. Taking a broader well-informed overview of life creates a healthier mental attitude. Surely it's better to live for the day, to take an interest in current affairs and to be generous in your opinions? It helps bridge the generation gap. Young people have a lot to learn from the experience and wisdom of us older people. They respect seniors who are not bigoted, opinionated and dismissive of youth.

Of course, if it's your brain that you want to train then you are never too old to sign up for a course at the Open University. At least 11 per cent of their students are over 50 and 3 per cent are over 60, and the number is growing all the time. Most older students opt for recreational courses, such as art history, but there are other choices including classical studies, English, history, philosophy, music and religious studies. If you are still working, then there are training courses available too.

Studying is good for the over-60s for many reasons, and not only for keeping up skills needed in the workplace. Learning will keep your brain active, will keep you in touch with the world around you and will give you the opportunity for socialising with other students. It is also another way to deal with the possibility of isolation, loneliness and depression that can accompany older age.

Get on the move, now!

Join the many older people who are healthier, more active and more involved in society than previous generations. Far from sitting down and taking life easy, these people are likely to be on the move. Some are off seeking adventures abroad; others are going back to university to improve their education, or bravely contemplating setting up new business ventures. Being active benefits your health as well as providing you with social contact to lift your spirits. It's time to 'sod sitting' and 'get moving!' Walking is an easy and efficient way to keep yourself in good health *and* shape. It boosts energy levels, gets the circulation going and makes your complexion glow. When you walk briskly, swing your arms, and puff a bit, this 'aerobic' exercise will increase your heart rate, lessening the risk of heart disease. It also encourages more oxygen into your lungs, improving your cardio-vascular system. Walking expends energy (calories), burns up fat and helps control your weight. Because walking is a 'weight-bearing' exercise (your body weight is supported by your spine, legs and feet), it helps maintain strong bones and build strong leg muscles, vital for your physical independence.

Perhaps you are a team player and relish the company of others? A game of golf combines walking, the skill of the game and social contact. Or why not join a sports club with facilities such as tennis, badminton, indoor and outdoor bowling, where you can meet like-minded friends? I belong to the U3A (University of the Third Age), a self-help group for those no longer in full-time work that provides educational, creative and leisure opportunities. The U3A also facilitates walking and rambling, and encourages activity holidays, all of which keep you fit while having fun. To join the 383,795 members in 999 U3As throughout the UK, look on the website www.u3a.org.uk and search the map by town or postcode for a branch near you. The membership secretary of the local U3A will give you details of what activities there are in your local area.

Why not join a gym? Many offer classes specifically for seniors, and a good discount rate. If you can afford it, a fully qualified and insured personal fitness trainer could encourage you to look after your body and motivate you to be more active in the privacy of your home. After an initial assessment a plan of action is drawn up, depending on physique, ability and personal requirements. The advantage of having a personal trainer is total flexibility; they will fit into your timetable

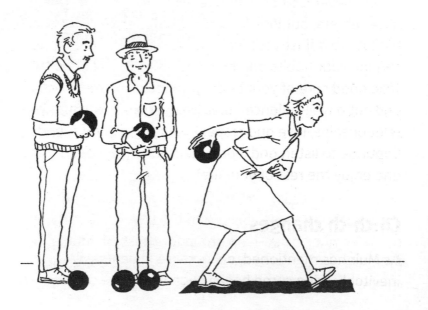

and you have the programme tailored to your level of fitness and physical abilities. Going at your own pace and under supervision, you can confidently build up your level of fitness. Ask them to use this book as your exercise reference guide. Or be your own personal trainer and take this book to heart – it's all here.

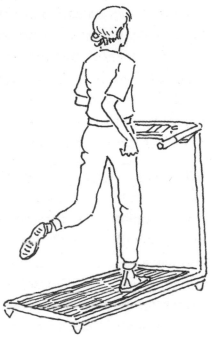

Feeling good is all about having a positive attitude to life. We should never look back and dwell on our failures or have regrets, but look forward with optimism. It's never too late to adjust your lifestyle, you're never too old to change your habits and help yourself to better health. Take good care of your body, your looks, be more active and eat a well-balanced diet (see page 42). Nurture your relationships, love and respect your family and friends. Continue to listen and learn, always keep an open mind and enjoy the rest of your life!

Ch-ch-ch changes

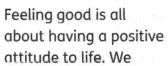

As Muir has mentioned, an increase in years will inevitably bring some bodily changes. There will be changes to your skeleton, with a natural thinning of bones in both men and particularly women. Changes occur in the joints; arthritis, rheumatism and backache are painful reminders of the passing years for too many people. With age, muscles can become weaker and less able to support your limbs – this is particularly true if you don't keep active. The muscles begin to atrophy, and your posture and self-esteem can be adversely effected by poor muscle tone.

There may be respiratory problems too for some older people, which are often brought about by insufficient exercise (and from the effects of smoking). These problems, in turn, decrease the efficiency of your cardio-vascular system (your heart and lungs), which can affect breathing and circulation, leaving you feeling fatigued and breathless. Sadly, too, there may be changes to your nervous system, which can result in memory loss, lack of co-ordination and balance.

Hereditary factors also play an important role in determining many of these changes, in just the same way as they can determine an individual's look and character. However, although some bodily decline is inevitable as the years pass by, much of the decline can be prevented, and some even reversed.

Exercise will keep you fit for work and play, and make you confident and more comfortable with yourself. For example, when you go travelling or are faced with an unexpected challenge, you feel able to cope. Exercise helps ease joint problems, and weight-bearing exercise (brisk walking etc.) can help prevent the bone disease osteoporosis. This is important as these conditions can restrict your mobility and rob you of your physical independence and quality of life in later years.

Modern grandparenting

It could be said that we mature folk are chronologically advantaged because we have so much to offer, not least of which is experience!

Many older people do age well and still have strong bodies, having regularly looked after their health over the years. We've certainly no control over our destined lifespan, but we do have some control over the quality of our lives. Growing older is inevitable, but it is not a disease, and today people are living longer thanks

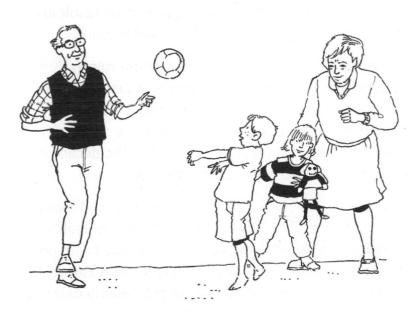

to medical advances and a better standard of living. Typically women in the UK today can expect to enjoy some 30 years more of life after menopause.

I am a granny. I'm called GG – an abbreviation of Granny Goddess, distinguishing me from other grannies! Grans today are confident women, juggling careers and home life. Most maintain their appearance, develop interests, are often financially and emotionally independent, and are interesting to know. Many expect to remain both physically and sexually active for many more years to come. However, too many grandmas and grandpas suffer from heart disease, stiff joints, osteoporosis, obesity and health-related problems, often caused by a lack of physical activity and poor diet. We also appear to be spawning a generation of couch potato children, many of whom won't be fit enough in their adult lives to support their parents, yet alone us, their sprightly grandparents in old age!

I have been blessed with four grandchildren (now young adults) who've made me acutely conscious of passing years and human fragility, highlighted 30 years ago as I coped with breast cancer. This taught me to appreciate and live life to the full. Good health is a major step to helping us overcome problems, enabling us to pursue ambitions, hopes and dreams. As the old Arab proverb says, 'He who has health has hope, and he who has hope has everything.'

And grandparents are likely to find themselves doing unusual things and sharing experiences with grandchildren they never thought possible at their age, activities usually reserved for parents. Many childish activities require stamina, and however fit, it's easy to find yourself exhausted by the exuberant energy of youngsters the second time around! I regard it as a privilege to be with my four grandchildren and look forward to special times from which I benefit emotionally. Wonderful, rewarding occasions! For distant grandparents it's well worth a journey, writing a postcard, sending an email or text to keep in touch with those children, family and friends we love.

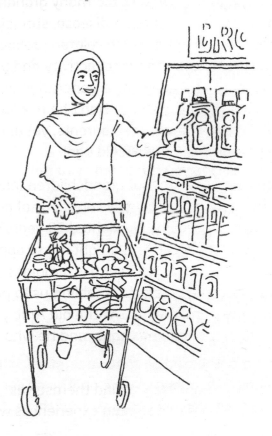

My nutrition action plan

Of course, exercise is not the only thing you can do to help yourself live well into your older years. Remember that it's also important that you eat a sensible well-balanced diet to keep healthy and in good shape. If you are what you eat, what stronger motivation do you need? Here are a few simple rules to follow when you are thinking about what to eat this week:

- Eat more fibre and less bad fat

- Consume more olive oil and less butter

- Shift from red meat to fish and chicken

- Eat at least five portions of fruit and vegetables a day, with more vegetables than fruit often has higher sugar content (fruit).

Eating a well-balanced and varied diet full of nutritious, fresh foods will give you the energy you need to do the things you enjoy, help maintain a healthy weight and keep you in good shape. A good place to start would be getting hold of a copy of Sod It! Eat Well by Anita Bean and Muir Gray, who recommend basing your diet on the Mediterranean diet, eaten by the world's healthiest people. The secret of their success is attributed to a combination of factors: an active lifestyle, low stress levels, strong family and community connections, and eating meals based on fruit, vegetables, whole grains, beans, fish, nuts and olive oil. The evidence is compelling. Researchers suggest that this eating pattern can protect against chronic disease, such as heart attack, stroke, cancer, type 2 diabetes and dementia, helping you live longer and making you feel happier.

Although there is no set 'menu' for a Mediterranean diet, here are 30 top tips for a healthy and balanced diet:

1. Eat more fibre-rich starchy foods – wholegrain breakfast cereals, wholemeal bread, pasta, brown rice, pulses, fresh fruit and vegetables

2. Cook vegetables lightly or stir-fry them – they retain their goodness when they're still crunchy

3. Snack on fresh and dried fruits, and unsalted (nuts which are higher in vitamins) *not* biscuits or chocolates

4. Use less sugar – less 'empty' calories

5. Choose sugar-free breakfast cereals

6. Cut down on saturated fats, found in butter, pies, cakes and biscuits, fatty cuts of meat, sausages and bacon, cheese and cream

7. Eat less red and substitute for while meat like poultry and fish

8. Avoid meat products like sausages, luncheon meat or salami

9. Full-fat milk is fine, but try skimmed and semi-skimmed as well

10. Foods such as butter, cream, fatty cheeses like Cheddar and Stilton, and also full-fat yoghurts should be eaten in moderation

11. Choose low-fat cheeses like Edam, Brie and cottage cheese

12. Eat more oily fish (but avoid frying it)

13. Throw out the chip pan and use the grill instead

14. If you fry food only use olive oil or rapeseed oil instead of vegetable or sunflower oil

15. Cut down on salt – we all consume more than we need

16. Avoid salty foods such as bacon, cheese, pizza, pickles, crisps, salted peanuts, savoury nibbles, and spreads such as Marmite and peanut butter

17. Use more seasoning, such as garlic, oregano and lemon juice, for flavouring

18. Drink 6–8 glasses of water a day

19. Drink herbal or fruit teas, which are caffeine-free and calorie-free

20. Drink a glass of sparkling water before meals to take the edge off your appetite, it may make you feel fuller

21. Cut out fruit juice (which is full of sugar), drink water or eat whole fruit instead

22. Opt for low-calorie drinks if you have to, but remember that water is a healthier option

23. Whisk an egg white with a carton of low-fat yoghurt or fromage frais for a creamy topping for a baked potato or fish

24. Instead of salad cream, make a light olive-oil-based dressing and use sparingly, or use natural low-fat yoghurt with lemon juice and herbs

25. Consider taking a vitamin D supplement (see next page)

26. Go easy on caffeine drinks like soda, tea or coffee late in the day, as they may prevent you getting a good night's sleep

27. Drinking too much alcohol may change the way you think and act, and could interact with your medical treatments (and is high in calories and sugar)

28. Avoid junk foods, takeaways, pies, pastries, margarines and cereal bars, which are high in fat and sugar, containing 'empty' calories and few nutrients

29. To lose weight eat more fibre-rich foods, eat less sugar, eat smaller portions and be more active

30. Finally ... sit at the table to eat (not in front of the telly), with family and friends if possible, eat slowly and chew your food thoroughly – that way, you'll stop eating when you're full

Physical activity is extremely important for maintaining bone strength and can also improve muscle strength, thus helping to prevent falls which can cause fractures. Calcium found in dairy products, such as milk, cheese and yoghurt, builds and maintains bone strength. Other good sources of calcium are green vegetables, tinned fish (eaten with the bones) and cereal products. But alongside the calcium, vitamin D is essential for maintaining bones and helping to prevent osteoporosis. Ideally we need 10 micrograms of vitamin D a day. Most of the vitamin D we use is formed in the skin by the action of summer sunlight between April and October. For some older people exposure to the sun can be limited and the ability to convert vitamin D to its active form is impaired with ageing. There is an increase in age-specific fracture risk related to a lack of vitamin D. Loss of muscle strength and reduced bone density contribute to falls and fractures, and the rates increase with age, so regular physical activity, such as walking, strengthens and builds up muscle and bone and increases calorie requirements. This in turn increases appetite and a more general sense of well-being. Because few foods contain vitamin D, I prefer to take a daily supplement of calcium plus vitamin D to ensure an adequate intake. These supplements are readily available at the chemist, where they can advise you on dosage.

My exercise plan

At the age of 77 I'm determined not only to get moving but to keep moving for as long as I possibly can. My 'Sod sitting, get moving' exercise plan consists of simple exercises specially designed for people who are largely neglected by the fitness industry. It's for those of us who are later on in life; those who haven't exercised in a while; and those who can't do the type of exercise they used to. It also involves a range of exercises specially designed for the less active to perform in the comfort of their living room, and even while sitting down.

GENERAL FITNESS TIPS

- Try to take half an hour of moderate physical activity five times a week

- Make exercise a natural part of everyday life and take the opportunity to be generally more active, anytime, anywhere

- Learn to breathe deeply in order to encourage oxygen intake and lung elasticity

- Stretch out your muscles before and after an exercise session or physical activity

- Take a brisk walk for at least half an hour each day

The 'Sod sitting, get moving' exercise plan consists of a head-to-toe warm-up, muscular core strength and endurance exercises plus a relaxation section. Stability drills help strengthen limbs and promote flexibility, while light aerobic work improves cardio-vascular capacity and circulation.

It's a fact that sitting for too long can result in slack abdominal muscles and slumped posture, which encourages cramp and indigestion. Inactivity is bad for our hearts and circulation, and often results in swollen legs and feet. Unsightly varicose veins are worsened by sitting with legs crossed at the knee and can be avoided by crossing them at the ankles instead. About half the UK population suffers from some kind of leg problem and about a quarter seek treatment for conditions such as varicose veins or leg ulcers.

Good circulation is important in preventing problems. When we exercise, blood that flows into the lower leg is helped back to the heart by the calf muscles acting as a pump, and by the one-way valves in our veins. However, if the veins become damaged or the valves stop working properly, blood can gather in the lower limbs, causing some people to experience problems such as swollen ankles and tired, aching legs.

THE BENEFITS OF EXERCISE – IMPROVING THE FOUR 'S'S

1. Stamina – gives you the energy to keep going

2. Strength – helps builds strong muscles to tackle any necessary work

3. Suppleness – encourages flexibility letting you to bend and stretch

4. Skill – being active encourages co-ordination of body and mind

    (There is a fifth S: Shape – exercising expends energy (burns calories) helping control your weight – which is an important bonus).

Before beginning the programme of exercises it is important to stress that you should be responsible for ensuring how suitable any exercise is for you. Everybody's health issues, especially those in the over-60 age group, are variable. Some people will be fitter than others, some stronger, others less flexible and some less stable.

Exercise should be comfortable and fun, and to get the most out of exercising try to join a class for older people. Most sport centres have qualified instructors who specialise in classes for the over-60s and those less mobile.

Exercise is not without its risks. To reduce the risk of any injury and/or illness, before beginning this or any exercise programme, please seek medical advice for guidance regarding appropriate exercise levels and precautions. It is particularly important to seek such advice if you suffer from an ongoing medical condition that may be affected by exercise. Special precautions are needed after surgery. Take extra care if you have had a hip replacement.

Always start any exercise programme slowly; never force or strain. While exercising, if you experience pain in your joints or muscles, stop, check your position and try again. If you feel any soreness, strain, discomfort, experience chest pain, dizziness or severe shortness of breath, stop immediately. If the pain persists seek medical advice and contact your GP. Remember: where there is pain and strain, there is no gain.

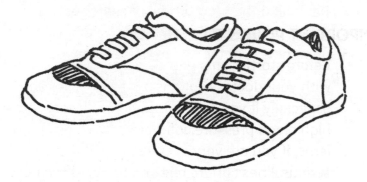

Wear comfortable clothes and supportive footwear.

Equipment you may need

You'll probably find most of these things around the house anyway, and you don't need to worry about buying anything unless you really want to do a particular exercise that uses something you don't have to hand.

- Sturdy trainers
- Mat
- Small pillow

- Upright armless chair

- Two small water bottles or light hand weights

- Exercise (resistance) bands

- Small soft ball (e.g. a tennis ball)

- 12-inch ruler or small stick

- Small bag of marbles

IMPORTANT POINTS TO REMEMBER

- Before starting any exercise programme check with your doctor that it is appropriate for you, especially if you suffer from heart disease, have high blood pressure, joint problems, back problems, if you are very overweight, if you have a serious illness or are recovering from an illness or operation.

- The 'Sod sitting, get moving' exercise plan is not a competition, so start slowly and build up gradually. If a movement hurts or you are suffering from dizziness – stop! Do what you can today and try again tomorrow.

- Check out location and surfaces before performing any exercises in your home or out in the garden.

- Clear a space and check that surfaces are not wet or slippery. Ensure that the support and equipment you use is strong enough to take your weight.

- Make sure you are warm enough: wear layered, loose clothing, which can be discarded as you warm up.

- Don't exercise for at least an hour after meals, and keep drinking water to avoid becoming dehydrated.

2

'SOD SITTING, GET MOVING!' EXERCISE PLAN

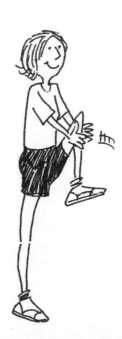

This chapter contains over 90 exercises to get you moving. If you are new to exercise or are not sure where to start, please see page 173 for my essential 5-a-day exercise plan to ease you in.

Part 1: Get moving, wake up and stretch

Your daily routine should be a mixture of standing, moving, sitting and some moderate aerobic exercise. Our exercise plan will help you maintain your physical independence and keep your body supple as the years pass. Make your workout last for a minimum of 10–15 minutes. The less fit you are, the longer you will need to warm up. All your movements should be rhythmic, not jerky. Doing any exercise to music of a medium speed can make it more enjoyable. Start your exercise session EVERY DAY with this great wake up and stretch.

Before you attempt any of these exercises, it's a good idea to read them through carefully so that you can visualise the movements. That'll save you having to stop and have another look midway through the exercise. It will also help you decide which exercises you want to do and whether they are suitable for you or not.

1. WAKE UP MONKEY STRETCH

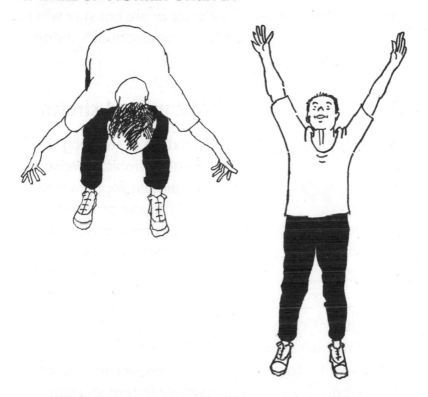

To stretch out the entire body: stand with your feet shoulder-width apart, bend the knees, bend forwards from the waist and swing your arms down to the floor and behind you. Now, in a flowing movement, straighten your knees, and swing your arms forwards and high above your head. Breathe deeply, lift your rib cage, straighten up and stretch your entire body. Repeat rhythmically five times.

> **Warning: Take extra care with this exercise if you have neck problems.**

2. BRIGHT EYES

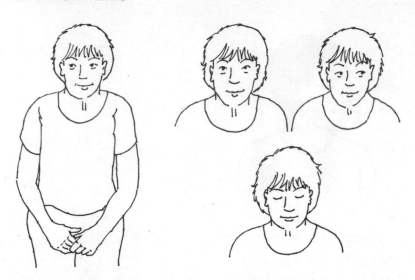

To relieve tension headaches and give your eyes a treat: sit or stand as in exercise 1 and look straight ahead. Without moving your head, use your eyes only to look first to the right and focus, now down and focus, then to the left and focus. Finally look up and focus. Repeat these simple movements five times.

3. HEAD ROLL

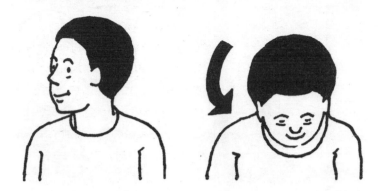

To release tension and mobilise the neck: look over your right shoulder with your chin parallel to the floor. Drop your chin to your chest and *slowly* roll your head to look over your left shoulder. Roll your chin back to your chest and move your head over to the right. Repeat five times with control. Do not roll your head backwards.

4. CHICKEN NECK

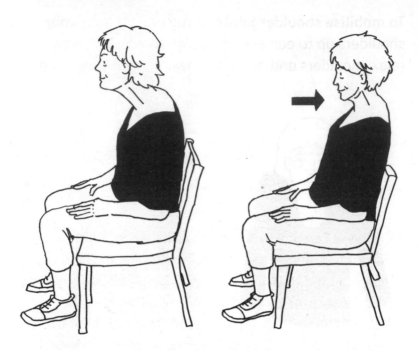

Release tension with this simple exercise: sit or stand upright with shoulders back, look straight ahead and stick your chin out forwards as far as you can. Keep your chin parallel to the floor. Now retract and pull your chin back hard, into your neck and upper chest. Stick your chin out again, parallel to the floor and then pull back hard. Repeat this chicken-like movement five times. It is excellent for posture and helping to prevent osteoporosis in the upper spine.

5. SHOULDER LIFT

To mobilise shoulder joints: shrug and lift both your shoulders up to ear level, or a high as possible. Now relax shoulders and press downwards with your hands.

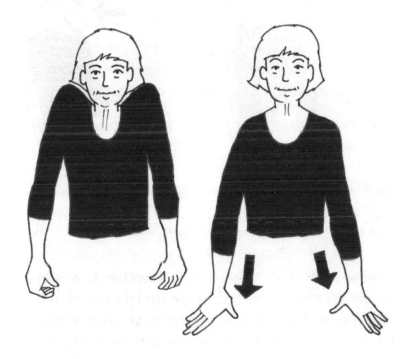

Part 2: Upper body, shoulders and back

The pace of modern life, the pressure of work and problems at home regularly cause tension headaches and often result in poor posture. We appear to carry the world on our shoulders, and many people will experience stiff necks and backaches as the years increase. Bad posture might also be due to badly designed chairs, a poor sitting position or too much sitting down in front of the TV or computer screen.

It is important to sort this out as soon as possible. There are some simple tricks you can do. Help yourself by checking that your chair, desk and worktop are at a good height and in sufficient light. Then check your posture. If you are working or relaxing, sit with your bottom well back on the seat. If there's an arch between your back and the chair then support it with a cushion or towel. Have your legs slightly apart, knees bent to an angle of 90 degrees with feet flat on the floor (if you've got short legs, a foot rest or block solves the problem). Poor posture can cause many problems: breathing becomes more difficult and the amount of air inhaled is reduced. For this reason it's important to maintain strength and mobility of the chest and back as we get older.

For seated exercising, always choose a firm upright chair (preferably without arms). Shuffle your bottom to the front of the seat and sit upright with your feet flat on the floor. Be aware of your posture and try to maintain a good position throughout the exercises.

6. SHOULDER CIRCLES

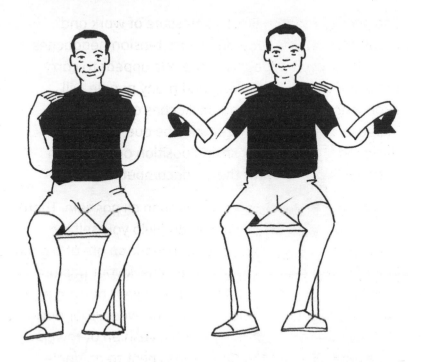

To release tension in your shoulders and upper back:
seated with your fingertips on your shoulders bring your
elbows together in front of your chest, then out to sides
and continue circling, pulling shoulder blades together.

7. SIDE REACH AND STRETCH

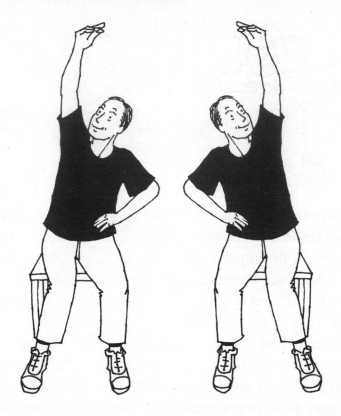

To improve the mobility of your shoulders and upper back: sit or stand with your feet shoulder-width apart. With your right hand, reach up and over your head as if climbing a rope (relax your left knee if standing). Hold the position for five seconds. Bring your right arm down and reach up and over with your left hand (relaxing your right knee) and hold the position for ten seconds. Repeat five times to each side.

8. SIDE TWIST

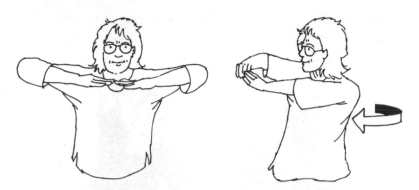

To improve the mobility of your shoulders and upper back: stand or sit upright as before but concentrate on posture by pulling in your tummy. Bend your elbows out, bring your hands up and touch your fingertips together in front of your chest. Keeping your elbows up, twist from your waist only and take your upper body, arms and head to look around your right side (as far as comfortable). Come back to the centre and continue to twist your arms and upper body to look around to your left side. Keep your elbows up, fingertips touching and repeat this twisting movement five times to each side, working the back and shoulders.

9. STANDING CHEST STRETCH 1

To stretch out your chest: place your hands on your bottom, bring your shoulders back together and stretch out your chest. Hold for ten seconds.

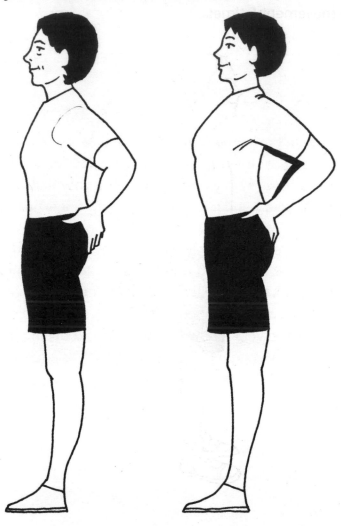

10. LIFT AND STRETCH 1

To expand the chest: sit or stand as already indicated. Clasp both hands behind your back. Lift and stretch both arms up behind you. Hold for ten seconds. Repeat the movement 5 times.

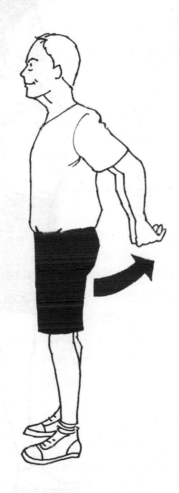

11. ARMS BACK

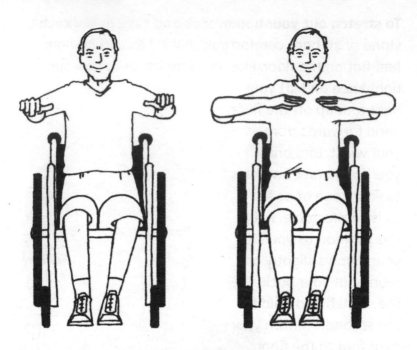

To improve mobility of shoulders and upper back:
stand or sit upright in your chair, face the front with
elbows up and fingertips together – remember your
posture. Keep your elbows up at shoulder level then
open your arms taking your hands out to the sides,
pulling shoulder blades together as far as possible. Keep
your elbows slightly bent – don't straighten or hyper-
extend your arms, and stretch out your chest. (Don't
poke your head forwards.) Bring your fingertips back
together in front of your chest. Repeat the movement
five times, breathing deeply throughout.

12. BACK STRETCH

To stretch out your upper back and relieve backache:
stand or sit back comfortably in your chair with your feet flat on the floor. Place both hands around your right knee and lift your right foot up off the floor. Bend forwards from your waist, and bring your forehead down on to your knee or as far as is comfortable. Keep this position as you lift your elbows slightly and round out your back. Feel the stretch and hold for ten seconds. Return your right foot to the floor. Repeat the movement, lifting your left foot and knee up, and holding the stretch for a further 10 seconds.

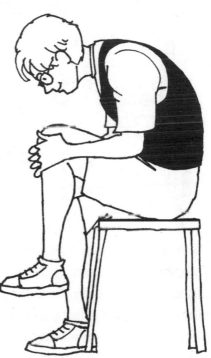

13. THE FLYER

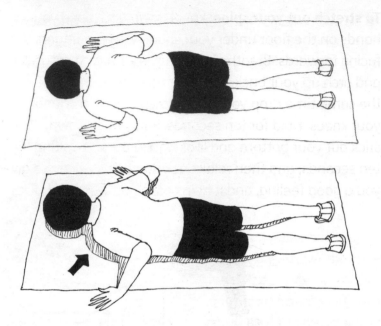

To strengthen your spine: lie on the floor on your tummy. Take your arms out to your sides. Bend your elbows and place your hands on the floor, palms down, under your shoulders. Keep your chin on the floor and breathe in. Keep your head, chest and arms in a *straight line* as you breathe out and lift them up together off the floor ... like a flying bird. Keep looking down (don't throw your head back). Breathe out and relax down. Repeat five times. It's a small but strong movement, so build up slowly.

Warning: This exercise is not suitable for those who suffer from osteoporosis.

14. THE CAT

To stretch out your spine: kneel down and place your hands on the floor under your shoulders with fingers facing forwards. Breathe in, pull up your tummy muscles and arch up your back (like a cat does on waking); at the same time drop your head down to look through your knees. Hold for ten seconds. Relax back down, stick out your bottom and look up. Hold that position for ten seconds, and then relax back down. This exercise gives you a good feeling, and it helps ease out that stiff back.

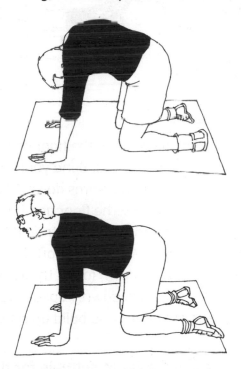

Warning: This exercise is not suitable for those who suffer from osteoporosis.

15. REST AND RELAX

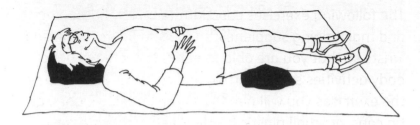

To relax your spine: lie down on your back and support your head with a small cushion. Place another small cushion behind your knees and thighs. Place your hands comfortably on your tummy. Breathe in deeply, taking the breath into your abdomen. Feel the rise and fall of your tum with your fingers. Close your eyes. Continue breathing deeply and relax for a few minutes. Take care getting up off the floor. Turn on to your side, then push yourself up on to one knee and carefully stand up.

Part 3: Arms, chest and wrists

The following exercises concentrate on strengthening and maintaining suppleness in the shoulders, arms and wrists so that you are able to perform everyday upper-body activities such as lifting and carrying. For some of the exercises you will need two small hand weights, or tin cans, or small plastic bottles filled with water or sand. You will also need a small soft ball (a tennis ball, for example) and 12-inch stick or ruler.

16. BICEPS – THREE OF A KIND

To strengthen front arm muscles/biceps: sit or stand with feet shoulder-width apart and tuck your elbows tightly into your waist. With palms uppermost, hold hand weights or small, filled plastic bottles out in front of you at waist level. Keep your elbows tucked in tight throughout the exercise, and simply lift the weights to your shoulders and lower them back out in front of you ten times with control. Then take the weights to your shoulders and then lift them up high and back down to your shoulders ten times. Finally take the weights to your shoulders and straighten your arms out in front of you ten times.

The triceps muscles at the back of your arms work with the biceps muscles in the front to produce strength and movement. Arms are prone to flabbiness as the years advance, especially if you have had a dramatic weight loss through dieting. If they are not exercised regularly the triceps muscles can become floppy.

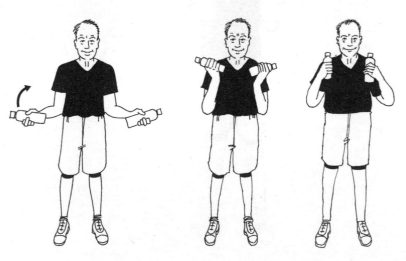

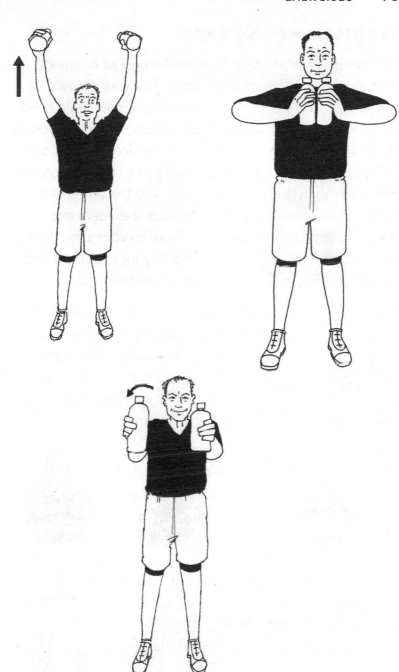

17. TRICEPS – ANTI-BATWINGS

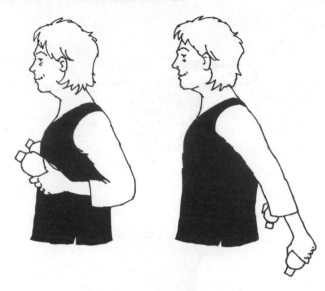

To firm up backs of your upper arms/triceps: sit or stand holding weights or bottles as before. Pull in your tummy to maintain good posture. Bend your elbows, holding the weights up at chest level, pull your shoulders back together and tuck your elbows into your waist. *Hold your upper arms in this position throughout the exercise.* Now straighten your lower arms only; take them down and back behind your body (turn your fists backwards at the same time). Now bend your elbows and bring the weights back up to chest level again. If you keep your upper arms steady with your elbows tucked in throughout the exercise you'll feel those back arm muscles working as you exercise. Repeat ten times to strengthen your triceps and tighten up those flabby 'batwings'.

18. FLINGS

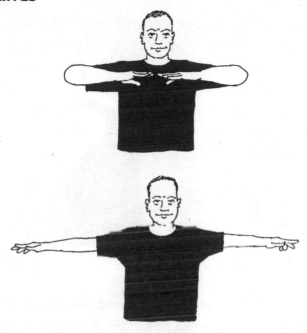

To tone up arms and expand chest: stand or sit.
Raise your arms up to shoulder level in front of your
chest, touch your fingertips together, palms down and
elbows bent. Part your fingertips, push your arms and
shoulders back once with a strong firm movement,
expanding your chest. Now open your arms wide and
fling your hands back once (*palms down*). Work your
upper back, bringing your shoulder blades together and
expanding your chest. Repeat the routine ten times,
going back to the starting position between each fling.
Wait a moment, then push back once more and fling
your arms open again, this time turning your palms
uppermost. Repeat the routine ten times.

19. TRICEPS STRETCH

To stretch out triceps muscles: sit or stand. Bend your right elbow, take your right arm up and place your right hand on your upper back. Take your left hand across your chest and push your right upper arm and shoulder back as far as possible. Hold for ten seconds. Then repeat the movement with your left arm and hold for ten seconds.

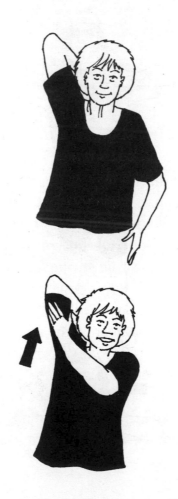

20. PALM PRESS

To strengthen wrists and arms: sit or stand. Bend your elbows and bring your arms up to shoulder level, palms together in the prayer position. Keep your fingertips touching but open out the palms of your hands. Now close palms by pushing wrists together hard. Continue opening and closing ten times. A small but effective exercise.

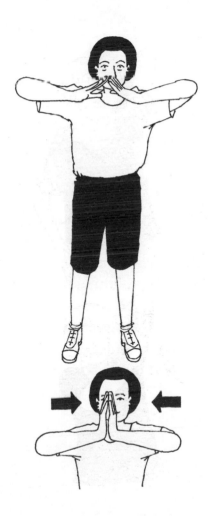

21. CUFF UPS

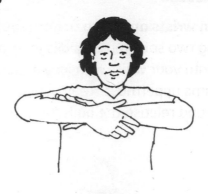

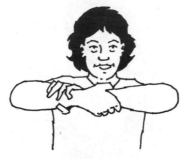

To work upper arms and chest muscles: stand or sit. Raise your arms up to shoulder level. Bend your elbows and, turning your hands, grasp the opposite arms firmly at wrist level. With short, firm movements 'push up' imaginary cuffs from each wrist. Feel the chest muscle jump and the underarm muscle work. Repeat ten times. This is an effective isometric exercise (in which you pit one muscle or part of the body against another to stretch it).

22. PALM SQUEEZE

To strengthen wrists and keep fingers supple: sit or stand. Holding two soft (tennis) balls (or oranges), tuck your elbows into your waist with lower arms out in front, and palms uppermost. Keep your arms and wrists still. Squeeze and release the balls ten times, as tightly as possible.

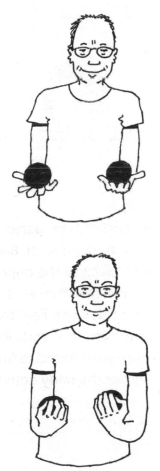

23. WIND UP

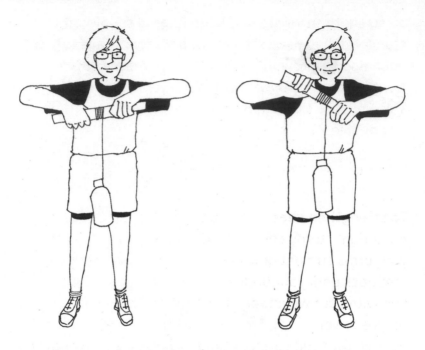

To strengthen your wrists: sit or stand. For this exercise you will need a stick or a ruler (approx. 1 inch across) and some string. Tie a piece of string 2–3 feet long securely in the middle of the stick. Attach a small but heavy object (for example, a plastic bottle filled with water) to the end of the string. Hold the stick at both ends with the palms of your hands facing downwards. Wind the string up with a twisting action. Reverse the action by holding the stick palms upwards and unwind with control. Repeat five times.

24. CHAIR PUSH UPS

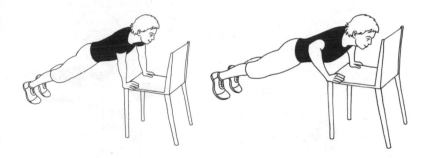

To strengthen chest, arms and wrists: stand facing
an upright sturdy chair placed against the wall. With
your arms straight grip the seat of the chair. Step your
feet back until your body and legs are in a straight
line with your weight on arms and wrists and at right
angles to your body. From this push up position bend
your elbows and carefully lower your upper body down
towards the chair seat. Now straighten arms and push
back up to start position with arms fully extended.
Repeat 10 times.

25. LIFT OFF

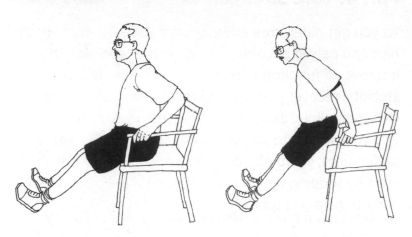

To strengthen your wrists and arms: sit forwards in an armchair. Extend your legs straight out in front with your heels to the ground and your toes pointing upwards. Place your hands, with fingers facing forwards, flat on to the arms of the chair. Incline your chest forwards (this corrects your centre of gravity) and try lifting your bottom off the seat. Take your body weight on your hands. Keep your legs straight and continue to lift and lower back down ten times. (If this is difficult, sit back into chair, and with bent knees repeat lifting and lowering, until your wrists become stronger.)

Part 4: Core strength, tums and bums

As you get older, core exercises (for your stomach, back, hips and pelvis) become very important because they improve all functional movement, increase balance and stability, recover posture and reduce the risk of falling. One marvellous extra is that they help you fit back into your favourite pair of trousers. Fancy that? OK, it's action time, so up off your bottom, and let's make a start by shaping up your seat. You will need an upright chair to help you tone up.

26. BALLET

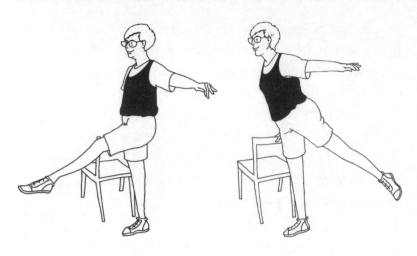

To work legs and bottom (gluteals): stand sideways to an upright chair, hold on with your left arm for support ... Stretch out your right arm like a ballet dancer, for balance. Point toes and swing your right leg forwards and backwards, working the muscles of thigh, hip and bottom. Continue ten times. Turn around to hold the chair with your right arm and swing your left leg as high as possible. Continue ten times.

27. BOB AND LIFT

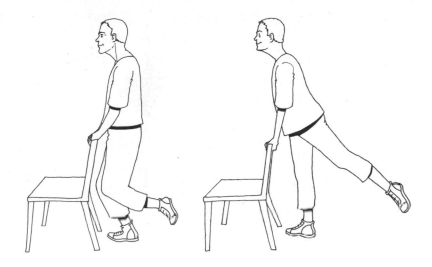

To work bottom muscles: stand facing the back of a chair and hold on with both hands. Slightly bend your right knee. Now lift your left foot up off the floor. Straighten your right knee, standing up; at the same time, straighten out your left leg behind you, pointing your toes. Hold up for five seconds. Repeat five times and feel your bottom muscles working. Repeat five times on the other leg.

Now it's time to get down to the bottom of the problem with some floor exercises to strengthen your bottom and your back.

> **Warning: Take care attempting these exercises if you suffer from back problems.**

28. KICKBACKS

To strengthen your bottom and your back muscles:
kneel comfortably with your hands on the floor,
shoulder-width apart. Drop your head down and lift your
right knee forwards and up to touch your forehead (or as
near as possible). Pull in your stomach and arch up your
back. With a smooth movement, look up and, at the
same time, straighten your right knee, stretch back and
hold for five seconds. Return to your original position.
Change knees and continue with your left leg, holding
for five seconds. Repeat five times with alternate legs.

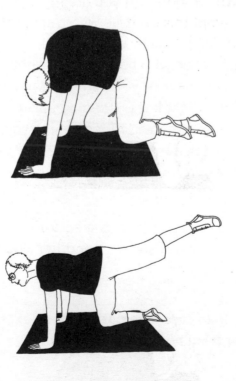

29. HIGH LIFTS

To tone and tighten bottom and thigh muscles (quadriceps): kneel down; bending your elbows, place your lower arms flat on the floor, hands together. Bend forwards to rest your head on your hands (you could use a small cushion for comfort). Pull up your tummy muscles but don't let your back sag. Take your left leg back, bending the knee 90 per cent. Keep your thigh parallel with the floor. With small, but controlled movements, bob your bent leg up and down ten times. Keep both hips facing downwards and feel your bottom muscles working. Change legs and bob your right leg up and down ten times. (If you are really fit you might want to attempt this exercise with a straight leg.)

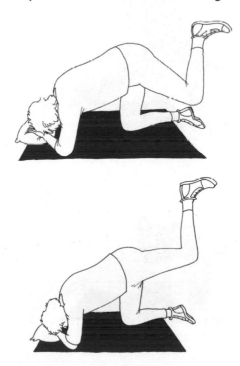

30. SIDE LIFTS

To work your gluteal (bottom) muscles: still kneeling, place your hands on the floor under your shoulders. Bend and lift up your left knee, gently taking it out to the left side. Hold your knee up parallel to the floor. Now, pointing your toes, straighten your left leg out to the side, working the hip and thigh muscles. Keep your left knee up, and repeat bending and straightening your leg ten times. Repeat ten times with your right leg.

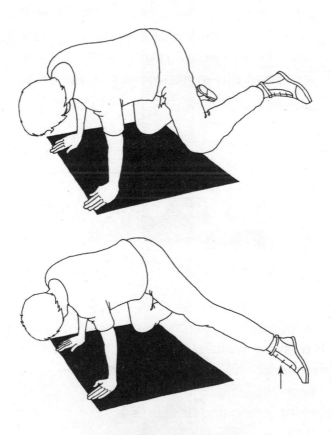

31. BOTTOM LIFT

To work your hips, thighs and bottom: lie back on the floor, arms at your sides, knees bent and shoulder-width apart. Clench your buttocks, pull in your tummy. Tilt your pelvis forwards and lift your bottom off the ground, transferring your weight on to your shoulders. Hold for five seconds. Relax down and repeat five times

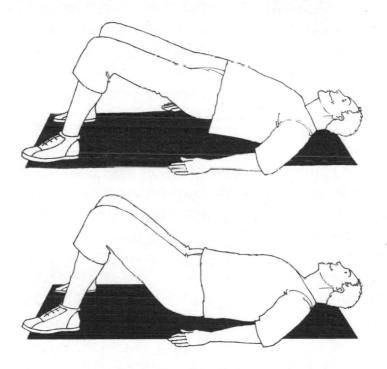

Before continuing to exercise the abdominal muscles, here is a simple exercise which I consider to be very important especially for women, to strengthen the pelvic floor (the sling of internal muscles which support the bladder, womb and back passage).

32. PELVIC FLOORS

To strengthen the pelvic floor: lie on your back, knees bent, feet slightly apart. There is no visible movement during this exercise. For women: first tighten the front passage (as if you are trying to stop spending a penny). Now tighten the vagina and finally the muscles in the back passage. Close your eyes and concentrate as you slowly pull up all the muscles at the same time. For men: pull up your back passage, at the same time try to stop an imaginary pee. Both hold for a count of five. Relax and repeat five times. Repeat this simple exercise anytime, anywhere to help prevent gynaecological, prostate and incontinence problems. It will also improve posture and help prevent backache.

Now it's time to strengthen our core (stomach, back, hips and pelvis) and tighten up those tummy muscles. Lie on the floor and support your head with a small cushion if uncomfortable. If you are a beginner you are allowed to 'cheat' for a few weeks while doing the next exercise by simply hooking your toes under the bed or sofa. This will also help protect a weak back.

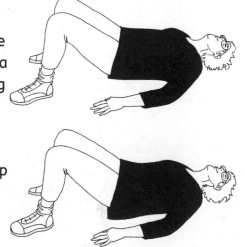

33. TUMMY TUCK

To strengthen abdominal (stomach) muscles: lie with
your knees bent and your feet flat on the floor shoulder-
width apart. Place your outstretched hands on your
thighs. Pull your tummy in, push your waist into the floor
and tilt your pelvis forwards (control and maintain this
pelvis tilt position throughout the exercise). Take a deep
breath in and as you breathe out, curl your upper body,
lifting your head and shoulders up as far as comfortable,
sliding your hands towards your knees. Breathe in again,
keep your back curled and, with control, slowly lower
yourself back down. Repeat the movement, building up to
ten times if possible. Don't let your head drop backwards
during the exercise. To increase the intensity, simply cross
your arms over your chest instead of placing them on
your thighs, or better still, by placing your fingertips to
your temples, keep your elbows out to the sides.

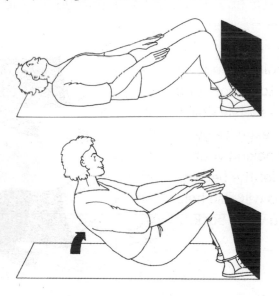

34. CRISS-CROSS

To strengthen the oblique stomach muscles (those on the sides of your body): lie as in the previous exercise but place your right elbow out on the floor and your right hand on your right temple. Pelvic tilt as before and breathe in. As you breathe out, lift your head and shoulders up and reach over with your left outstretched hand to touch the outside of your right knee. Breathe in, relax back and repeat to other side. Continue the exercise to alternate sides ten times.

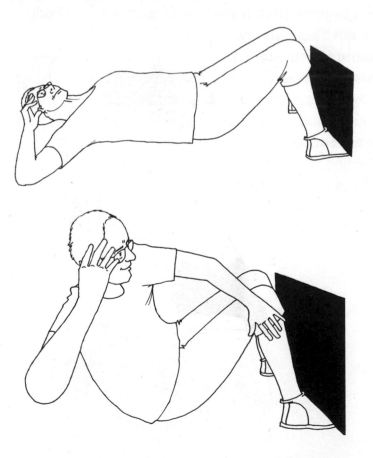

35. TUMMY STRETCH

To stretch out and relax stomach muscles: lie on the floor as before with your knees still bent but extend both arms out to your sides with palms facing down. Keep your feet in contact with the floor throughout. Breathe in and, as you breathe out, twist only from your waist to take your knees over to your left side to touch the floor (or as far as comfortable). Keep your shoulders down on the ground but turn your head to look over to the right as far as comfortable. Relax for ten seconds, enjoying the stretch you feel right across your body.

Breathing out slowly, return to your start position. Repeat, taking your knees to your right and looking over to your left. (Closing your eyes will add to the relaxation.)

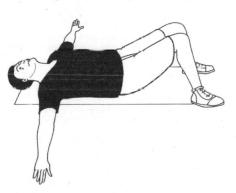

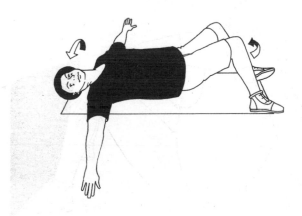

Part 5: Thighs, legs and feet

Are you on your feet for hours a day? When your legs and feet feel tired, have you noticed your whole body tends to feel tired and achy, and you slow down? It's as though your total well-being is dependent on the fitness of your limbs, and if your legs ache and ankles swell you may also have a tendency to varicose veins. Good circulation is important in preventing leg problems and strong legs are essential for mobility, so it is important to exercise them regularly to maintain strength. Women have naturally less leg power than men. Strong muscles provide stability and if we trip, strong muscles help correct our posture by supporting the bones and preventing fractures. You will need your mat, pillow, exercise bands and an upright chair for the following exercises.

Take care with these exercises if you have an existing back injury or if you have any difficulties with your balance. You should feel no pain ... but if in doubt leave it out!

36. HAPPY FEET

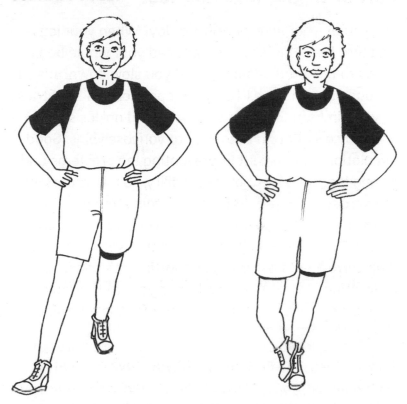

To mobilise your ankles and feet: stand and place your hands on your hips. Straighten out your right leg and place your right foot out in front of you with your heel down on the floor. Now bring your right foot back and touch your toes to the side of your left foot. Repeat the heel/toe action ten times. Change to your left foot and repeat ten times, keeping your supporting leg 'soft' (slightly bent).

37. ROCK AND ROLL

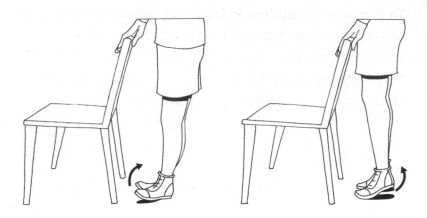

To increase circulation in the legs and maintain mobility of the ankles: stand, holding a chair for support, with your feet flat on the floor. Keeping both heels on the floor simply pull your toes and forefoot up towards your shins. Now, pointing your toes, lower them back down to the floor, then lift both heels up with a rolling action. Repeat rock and roll action as vigorously as you can fifteen to twenty times. Feel the strong pumping action in your calf.

38. ANKLE CIRCLES

To increase circulation in legs and improve mobility of ankles: stand as before. Lift your left foot off the ground and point your toes. Circle and rotate them (your ankle only, not your leg) first clockwise 15 times, then anti-clockwise 15 times. Repeat with the right foot.

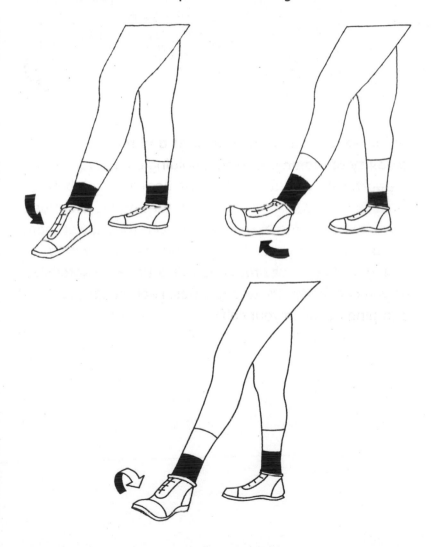

39. FRONT AND SIDE LIFT

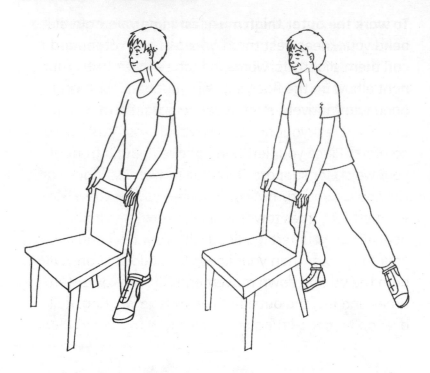

To strengthen the quadriceps (front thigh muscles):
stand and hold the back of a chair for support.
Straighten your leg, point your toes and lift your leg
high out in front and hold for five seconds. Keep your
leg as high as possible and take it on out to the side and
hold for five seconds. Relax your leg down and repeat
with the other leg. Repeat five times with each leg. Keep
your supporting leg 'soft' (slightly bent).

40. ABDUCTORS 1

To work the outer thigh muscles: lie on your right side, bend your knees, rest them on top of each other and curl them slightly forwards (banana shape). With your right elbow on the floor, support your head with your hand (alternatively, stretch out your right arm with palm down and rest your head on it with a small cushion for comfort). Place your left hand on the floor (in front of your waist) for support. Don't roll forwards or backwards. Now pull in your tummy and tighten your bottom. Flex your left foot (toes towards shin); keeping your knee bent, lift up your left leg (lead with your heel and keep your foot lower than your knee). Relax down. Controlling both the up and down movements, lift and lower ten times and feel the outside thigh muscle working. Roll over and repeat, lifting and lowering with the right leg.

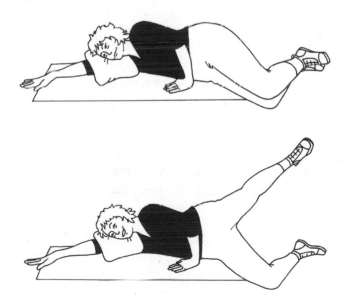

41. ABDUCTORS 2

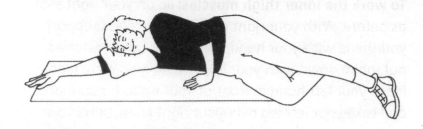

To increase the intensity of exercise to strengthen outer thigh muscles: lie down as in exercise 40. Flex your toes but straighten your top left leg and lift it up as high as possible, leading with your heel. Remember to keep your tum and bum tight throughout the exercise. Begin with ten lifts, then roll over on to your left side and repeat the exercise with a straight right leg. (You can add leg weights to increase the intensity still further.)

42. ADDUCTORS

To work the inner thigh muscles: lie on your right side as before. With your right elbow on the floor support your head with your hand (or straight arm stretched out, palm down with your head resting on a cushion). Place your left hand in front of your waist for support and take your left leg over your right knee. Bend your left knee and place it down on the floor. Now straighten out your lower right leg (in a straight line with your upper body) and flex your right foot. Lead with your heel, and lift and lower with short sharp movements, fifteen to twenty times. Feel the small inner thigh muscles working. Roll over to your left side, take your right knee over to the floor and repeat this 'pulsing' movement with your left leg fifteen to twenty times.

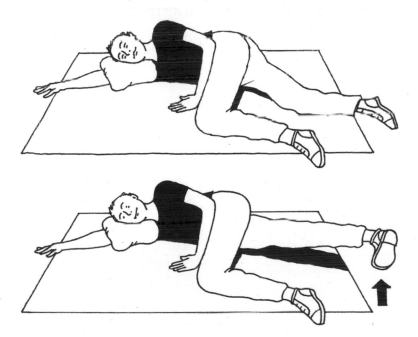

43. DOUBLE LEG LIFT

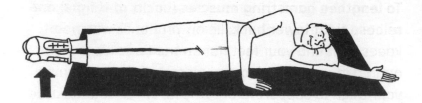

To strengthen abdominals and firm thigh muscles: lie down on your left side with one hip stacked on top of the other with your head resting on your stretched-out arm, palm up. Place your left hand on the floor in front of your waist for support, and slightly curve your legs forwards. Inhale, and as you breathe out lift both legs up about 10 centimetres from the floor, pressing them tight together. Hold for a count of five and repeat five times. Roll over to your right side and repeat another five times.

44. HAMSTRING STRETCH 1

To lengthen hamstring muscles (backs of thighs) and release tight lower back: lie on your back with your knees bent and your feet flat on the floor, hip-width apart. Lift your right leg and place your hands behind your thigh to support it. Breathe in; check your posture to protect your back (ensure your waist is pushed down into the floor and that your pelvis is tilted up). As you breathe out, pull in your tummy, straighten your leg and lift it up as high as possible. Flex your foot and hold for ten seconds. Carefully place your foot down on the floor and repeat with the left leg (you can use an exercise band around your foot if this is difficult for you).

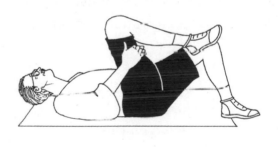

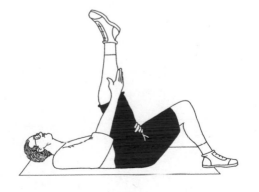

45. QUADS STRETCH 1

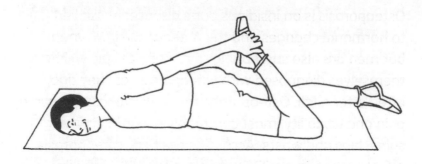

To stretch out quadriceps (front of thighs): roll over on to your tummy, keeping your head and shoulders down on the floor. Take your left hand and reach behind you, bend your knee and grasp your ankle (not your toes). Gently ease your foot towards your bottom (or as far as is comfortable) and feel the stretch in your front thigh. Hold for ten seconds. If you find this difficult, use an exercise band around your ankle and pull up towards your bottom as far as possible. Repeat with your right hand and ankle, and stretch out for ten seconds. (If you have trouble getting down on the floor, this stretch can be performed standing up, using an exercise band and chair back for support.)

Part 6: Bones and osteoporosis

Osteoporosis is an insidious bone disease. It is linked to hormonal changes and the menopause in women, but men are also susceptible to it. Many people will find themselves diagnosed with osteoporosis as they age, often after a fall. Osteoporotic fractures can cause severe pain and disability, most commonly occurring in the spine, hips and wrists. According the NHS, osteoporosis affects over three million people in the UK. Each year more than 500,000 people receive hospital treatment for fragility fractures (fractures that occur from standing height or less) as a result of osteoporosis. One in two women and one in five men over the age of 50 will have a bone fracture mainly as a result of this condition.

Results of published research show that osteoporosis is preventable in many cases, and that a healthy and active lifestyle can help guard against it and reduce the risk of falls and resulting painful fractures. It's not just about getting old, as was previously assumed. You can help keep your bones strong by doing regular weight-bearing exercise. That is any kind of physical activity where you are supporting the weight of your own body, such as, jogging, tennis and brisk walking.

The following unique exercises will help strengthen your bones by targeting the bones most at risk of sustaining osteoporotic fractures. These bone-strengthening exercises consist of easy movements designed specifically to strengthen and preserve bone thickness.

Aim to do a minimum of 10 minutes of exercise a day, three days a week, though I do ask that you build up slowly, to avoid possible injury or over-tiring. It is advisable to check with your doctor before commencing any exercise programme. If you have osteoporosis, it is advised that you lie down on the floor or a bed to perform the floor exercises and support your neck with a small cushion or towel. For those of you with vertebral fractures, painful, tender spines and limited mobility, some exercises may be too difficult. The upper back and foot exercises can be performed while sitting down.

You will need a wall or a sideboard for support, an exercise band or a hand towel, a 2 lb bag of sugar, a walking stick, a small cushion and an exercise mat for these exercises.

Warning: Do not attempt these exercises if you have advanced osteoporosis.

The following pages show exercises you can do in your everyday life: around your home, in the workplace or in the garden to strengthen ankles, hips and spine. Try this weight-bearing exercise to start: hold on to a worktop or the banisters, lift up your right leg, transferring your weight to your left side, and hop ten times. Turn around, lift up your left leg, transferring your weight to your right side and repeat, hopping ten times. If you can do that one, then you should be fine to press on.

The following two exercises can be done sitting in a chair to help keep ankles mobile.

46. FIDGETY FEET

To strengthen hips and ankles: sit or stand with your
feet slightly apart. Use a broom or walking stick and,
hold the top of it for support. Bend and pull your knees
inwards, lift your heels up pushing them outwards
and take your weight on your now inward facing toes.
Now keeping your body upright with your weight on
your toes, push your knees outwards, and with a small
bobbing action pull your heels together with your toes
now facing outwards. Repeat bobbing and turning your
feet working the ankles 10 times.

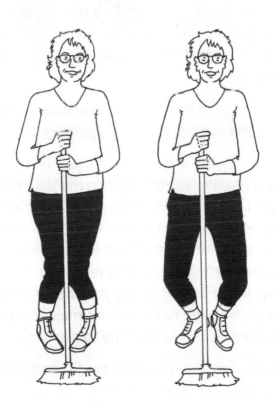

47. EDGY FEET

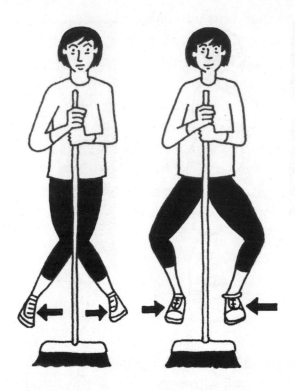

To strengthen hips and ankles: still holding your broom or walking stick for support, move your feet wider apart with your toes facing forwards. Bend and knock your knees together, taking your bodyweight on to your insteps. Keep your feet parallel and your body upright. Then, with a small bobbing action, take your knees out wide and transfer your weight on to the sides of your feet. Repeat ten times.

48. PUSH-AWAYS

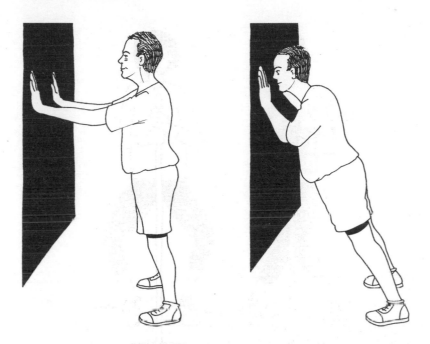

To strengthen wrists and arms: stand a foot or two away from a wall with your arms slightly outstretched. Have your feet apart and your arms up at shoulder level. Place your hands flat on the wall and incline your fingers inwards. Pull in your tummy, keep your head, neck and back in a straight line, bend your elbows out and lower yourself carefully towards the wall. Take your bodyweight on your wrists and hands but don't allow your body to sag. Now straighten your arms and push your body back upright. Repeat ten times. If possible, keep your heels down; you will stretch out your calf muscles (back of lower leg) at the same time.

49. PULL-AWAYS

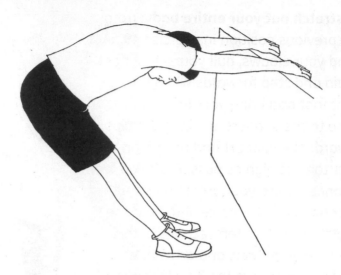

To strengthen wrists, arms and stretch out shoulders and spine: with your feet hip-width apart, stand a few feet away from a secure kitchen unit such as the sink or sturdy banisters. Bend forwards from the waist and hold on to the support securely with both hands. Keeping your legs straight, drop your head down and flatten out your back. Pull your body away from the support, taking the weight on your wrists, arms and shoulders. Hold the stretch for ten seconds.

50. REACH UP

To stretch out your entire body: from the previous position in exercise 49, bend your elbows, pull yourself upright again and step forwards with your right foot and bring your left to join it, close to the support. Incline your hips towards the support and rise up on to your toes as high as possible. If you feel balanced, raise your arms and stretch your hands up to the ceiling. Hold the stretch for five to ten seconds before lowering your heels and arms down. Heel raises correct the body's centre of gravity and improve balance, helping to prevent falls.

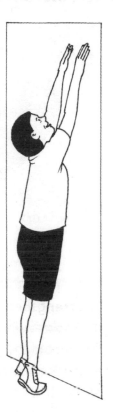

51. WRIST STRENGTHENER

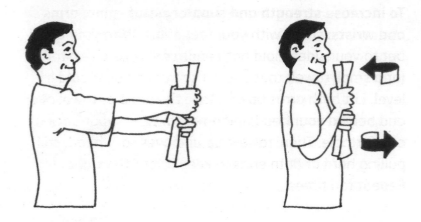

To help improve bone and muscle strength in hands and wrists: fold or roll an exercise band or small towel. Holding it with both hands, squeeze hard, then twist with your wrists, bringing your elbows close to your body. Hold for a slow count of five (and count out loud to ensure you don't hold your breath). Release and repeat ten times.

52. UP AND OVER

To increase strength and suppleness of spine, arms and wrists: stand with your feet apart. With your arms out to your sides, hold both ends of an exercise band (or a small towel) taut out in front of you at shoulder level. Lift both arms up and take the band or towel over and behind your head and on as far down your back as comfortable. Then, raise it up and over your head, still pulling hard at both ends to keep it taut throughout. Repeat ten times.

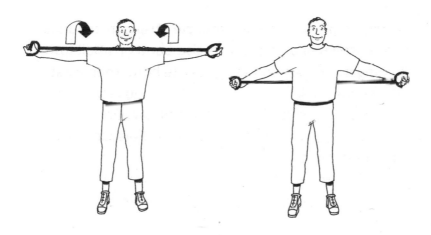

53. BACK RUB

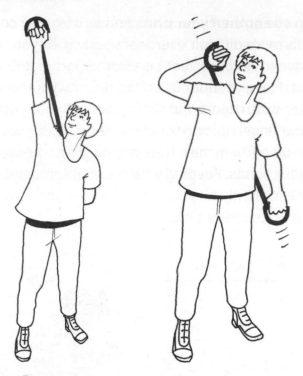

To help strengthen wrists and spine and increase mobility in your upper back: hold one end of an exercise band (or a small towel) with your right hand. Drop the other end over your shoulder and down behind your back. Reach behind your waist with your left hand and grasp the other end of the band. Pull it taut, by extending your right hand upwards. Keeping the band taut, pull it down with your left hand in a sawing motion. Repeat this sawing action ten times. Reverse your hands and repeat ten times.

54. BOTTOMS UP

To help strengthen your arms and wrists: take care with this more difficult exercise. Sit down on your mat with your knees bent, feet hip-width apart and flat on the mat. Place your hands on the floor by your sides, shoulder-width apart and slightly behind your bottom with your fingers facing forwards. Carefully lift your bottom up a few inches, transferring your bodyweight on to your hands. Keeping your body upright, push your chest slightly forwards and hold for five seconds if possible. Repeat five times.

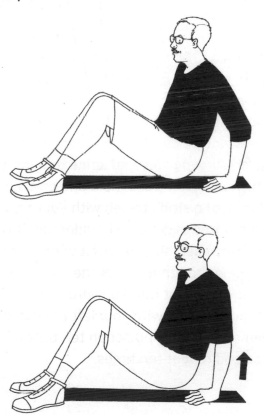

55. KNEES OVER

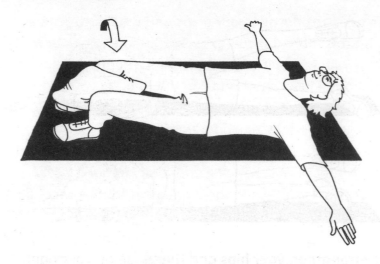

To mobilise hips, thighs and lower back: lie on your back, knees bent, feet flat on the floor and hands by the side of your bottom, palms down. Keep both feet and shoulders in contact with the floor throughout this exercise. Place a cushion (alternatively, if more advanced, a 2 lb bag of sugar) between your knees. Gripping the cushion/weight with your knees, roll them together over to the left side, as far as is comfortable. Relax for five seconds. Bring your knees back to centre then roll them over to the right and relax for five seconds. Repeat five times if possible.

56. LEG LIFTS

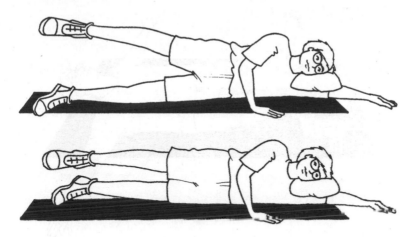

To strengthen your hips and thighs: lie on your right side, legs stacked together and out straight. Support your head with your right hand or rest your head on a cushion with your right arm outstretched. Place your left hand on the floor at waist level for balance. Raise your left leg up (not too high) and bring your right leg up to join it. Squeeze your thighs, knees, calves and ankles together and hold for five seconds. Repeat five times. Relax both legs down. Roll over and repeat the exercise on the other side.

Alternatively, if this is too advanced, lie out on your right side as before with both legs straight but then bend your right leg to stabilise your position. Lift up your left leg only and hold for five seconds. Repeat five times. Roll over, bend your left leg and lift your right. (Beginners may find it more comfortable to also bend the lifting leg.)

Part 7: Strength, balance and the prevention of falls

Having a good sense of balance helps us remain physically independent as we get older. It enables us to walk without staggering, bend over without falling, climb stairs without tripping and get up from a chair with ease. As we age, we are more likely to suffer issues with our balance, but these problems don't always occur because of age. For example, some balance disorders are caused by problems of the inner ear, when the labyrinth becomes infected or swollen (labyrinthitis). Low blood pressure can cause dizziness, and Ménière's disease of the middle ear causes vertigo, poor balance and hearing problems. Other balance disorders may be prompted by a head injury or a disorder in another part of the body, such as the brain or the heart. Diseases of the circulatory system, such as stroke, can cause dizziness, and smoking and diabetes increase the risk of stroke.

In many cases, however, you can help to reduce your risk of balance problems. Unsteady balance due to high blood pressure can be managed by eating less salt (sodium), maintaining a healthy weight and exercising. Some medicines, such as those taken to help lower blood pressure, can make a person feel dizzy. And if your medicine is ototoxic (literally 'ear poisoning') – as is the case for some antidepressants, sedatives, tranquilisers, diuretics, some analgesics (painkillers) and certain chemotherapeutics (anti-cancer drugs) – you may feel off balance. Other medicines too may disturb your balance, so check with your GP if you notice a problem. Ask if other medications can be used instead; if not, ask if the dosage can be safely reduced. Sometimes it can't be, but your doctor will help you get the medication you need while trying to reduce unwanted side effects.

The following exercise instructions and advice are in no way intended as a substitute for professional medical advice specific to any individual case.

You will need an exercise band and a bag of marbles for the following exercises (see Part 8 below for more details). In the meantime, you can use tea-towels or tights instead. Begin by ensuring that your upright, armless chair is suitably sturdy and stable.

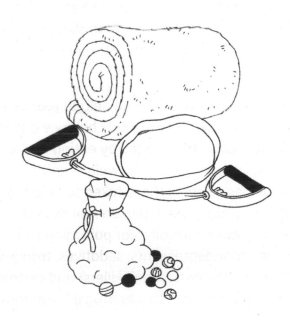

57. SIT TO STAND

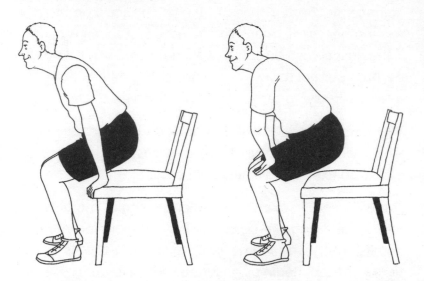

To strengthen your quadriceps (front of your thighs) and improve balance: sit tall near the front of the chair. Place your hands on your thighs and lean slightly forwards, with your feet slightly behind your knees. Stand up, using your hands on the chair seat to push up if needed (progress to hands on thighs as you get stronger over time). Take your feet back until your legs touch the chair, then stand up tall, bend your knees and slowly lower your bottom back into the chair. Repeat ten times.

58. PULL-BACKS

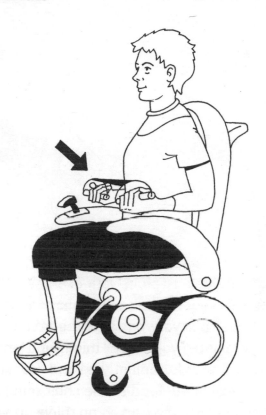

To strengthen arms, wrists and upper back: sit upright in your chair. Hold your exercise band with your palms facing up and wrists firm and straight. Pull your hands apart, then draw the band towards your hips and squeeze your shoulder blades together. Hold for a slow count of five (count out loud to keep breathing), then release. Repeat ten times.

59. PULL AND PUSH

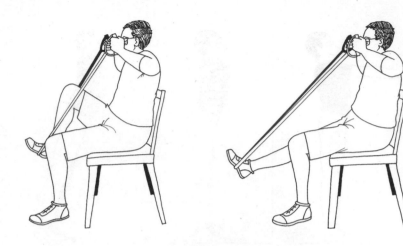

To strengthen the legs: place your exercise band under the ball of your right foot. Sit tall, lift your right knee a few inches, then pull your hands towards your hips and hold. Now straighten your right knee by pushing your foot firmly downwards against the band. Hold for a slow count of five (count out loud to keep breathing). Bend the knee and release the arm. Repeat five times, and then change to your left leg.

60. WALL PRESS-UPS

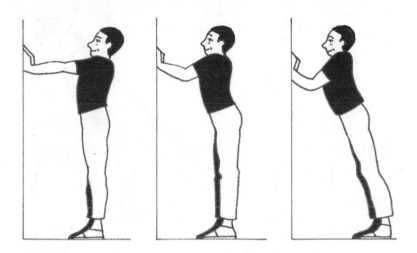

To strengthen wrists, arms, bottom and stretch the backs of your legs: stand an arm's length from the wall. Place your hands on the wall at chest height, fingers upwards. Keeping your back straight and your tummy tight, bend your elbows, lowering your body with control towards the wall. Press back to the start position. Repeat ten times. If find this easy, you can step further back from the wall, but remember to keep both heels down. Feel the stretch in the lower leg.

61. SIDE STEPS

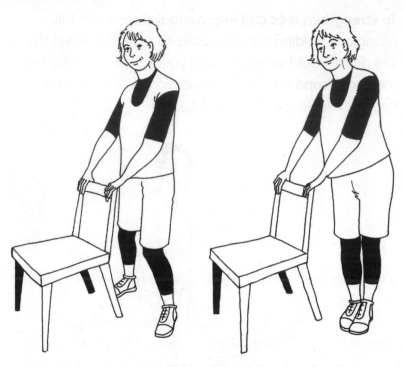

To encourage balance and stability: stand tall, holding the chair back with both hands. Move your right foot out to the side and then back to the centre. Then do the same with your left foot. Continue stepping from side to side for about a minute. When you're confident, try holding the chair with only one hand. Now try two steps to the side and back for one minute.

62. HEEL RAISES

To strengthen legs and improve balance: stand tall, facing and holding a sturdy table, chair back or even the sink. Raise your heels up, taking your weight over the big toe and second toe. Hold for five seconds. Lower your heels to the floor with control. Repeat ten times.

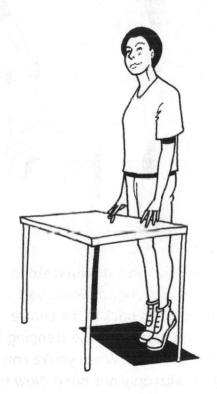

63. TOE RAISES

To strengthen legs and improve balance: stand tall, using a support as above. Raise your toes up towards your shins, taking your weight back on to your heels but without sticking your bottom out. Hold for five seconds then lower your toes to the floor with control. Repeat ten times.

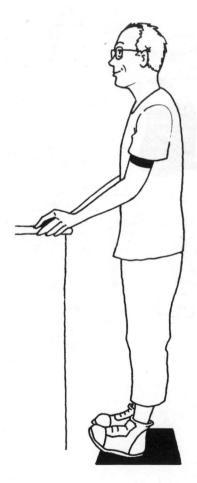

64. MARCHING

To improve stamina: stand to the side of the chair, holding on to it with one hand. Stand tall. March on the spot swinging your free arm. Keep marching for one minute.

Turn slowly around then repeat, marching using the other arm. Repeat five times.

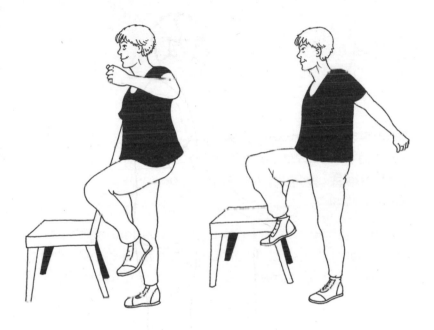

65. LEG SWINGS

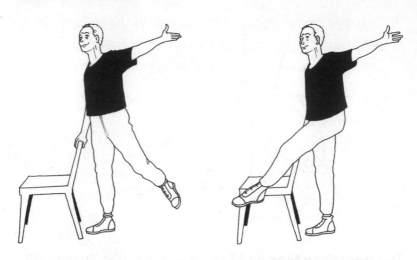

To improve hip mobility: stand to the side of the chair, holding on to it with one hand. Stand tall. Swing the leg furthest away from the chair forwards and back with control.

Perform ten swings (try not to lean over during the movement). Turn slowly around then repeat, swinging the other leg ten times.

66. TOE TIME

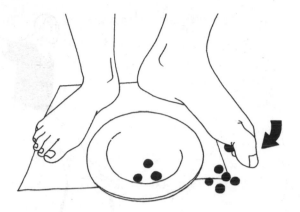

To strengthen toes and feet, and aid balance: you will need your bag of marbles for this one. Sit comfortably in a chair in bare feet. Place ten marbles on the floor (or mat) and an empty container in easy reach of your feet. Using your left foot, pick the marbles up one by one and release them into the container. Continue until all ten marbles are in the container. Repeat, picking up ten marbles with your right foot.

Part 8: Resistance band exercises

It struck me while compiling the exercises for this book that if you were going to take the trouble to buy a resistance band (also known as an exercise band) then I should include a section dedicated to them. They are available in supermarkets, sports shops and probably your local sports centre too.

Resistance bands are basically large elastic bands that you can use to exercise all areas of the body. I always buy the ones with handles on the ends, but you can get them without handles too. They can be good for people with limited mobility, as many of the exercises can be done while seated. They are not expensive and I would recommend you get some. However, if you don't want to buy one then you can use an old pair of tights or a small towel instead.

67. STAND AND CURL

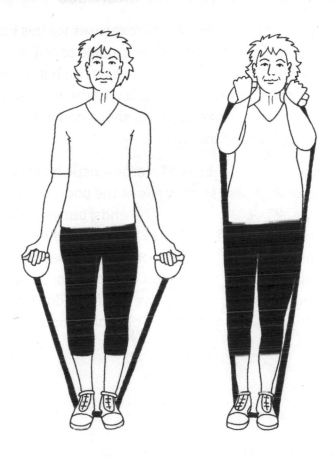

To strengthen your biceps: stand upright with both feet on the centre of the band, your feet slightly apart. With your arms at your sides, grip the band with your palms facing upwards. Bend your elbows and pull your fists up to your shoulders, then relax down. Repeat ten times.

68. V FOR VICTORY

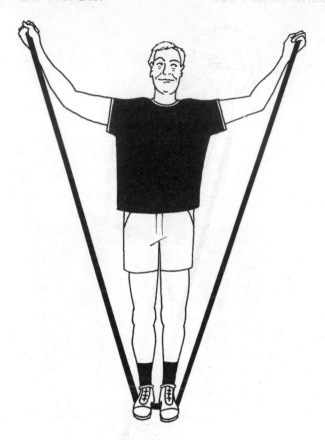

To strengthen shoulders and improve posture: stand with your feet slightly apart on the centre of the band. With your arms at your sides, grip the handles with palms facing in. Pull your shoulder blades together and raise your arms up and out to the side, then relax down. Repeat ten times.

69. BEND AND PULL

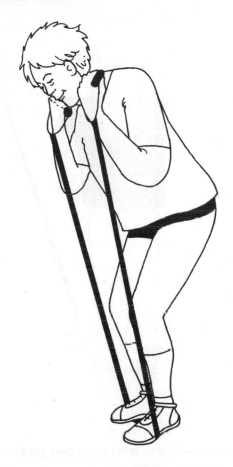

To strengthen arms and shoulders: stand as in exercise 67 with your arms at your sides. Grip the handles with your palms facing in. With soft knees, bend slightly forwards from the waist, stick your bottom out. Keeping your core muscles tight, bend your elbows and pull the bands straight up to shoulder level. Repeat ten times.

70. ROW THE BOAT

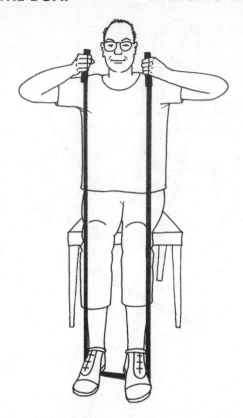

To strengthen arms and shoulders: sit tall with legs out straight. Place the band under the soles of your feet. With your arms straight out in front of you, hold the handles with your palms facing one another. Bend your elbows and pull the band towards your chest, squeezing your shoulder blades together in a rowing motion. Keep your core muscles tight throughout the exercise, then relax. Repeat ten times.

71. LIFT AND STRETCH 2

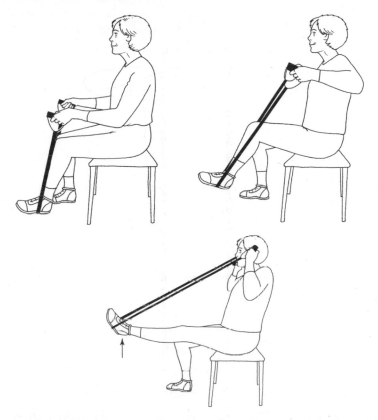

To strengthen legs: sit tall with your knees bent and your feet flat on the floor. Place the band under your right foot, holding the handles with your palms facing one another. Lift and straighten your left leg, pulling the band outwards up to shoulder level to work your leg. Keeping the band tight and your leg straight, continue lifting and lowering ten times but without touching your heel to the floor. Keep your core muscles tightened throughout the exercise. Repeat with your right leg.

Part 9: Chair exercises

I have devised a programme of chair exercises to encourage good balance and help prevent falls. As stated in the introduction of this book, they are in no way intended as a substitute for professional medical advice specific to any individual case. These simple chair exercises will revitalise your body, reoxygenate your system, and improve your circulation and digestion.

Reintroducing exercise into the lives of the less active is key to maintaining a sense of independence and quality of life for those who are getting older or are restricted in their movements. Working out isn't exclusively for the super-fit, but accessible to everyone whatever their age or level of fitness.

Sitting incorrectly for hours on end can result in skeletal and muscular problems, but helping yourself to better health with this 'Get moving' programme of seated exercises can add quality to your life. Even from the confines of your chair, give yourself a break, think about your posture and literally take a breather. For extra stability it is advisable that you place your feet on a small block or some books, and you hold on to the seat of your chair with your free arm during some of the movements and stretches. If you are able to stand and support yourself with the chair you will benefit even more, by simply moving and marching in time to the music. This will help strengthen your leg muscles and improve your balance.

SAFETY WHEN EXERCISING IN CHAIRS

- Use a sturdy, stable upright chair for support

- Wear comfortable clothes and supportive footwear

- Prepare a space and have your exercise bands, small water bottles or hand weights ready before you start

Take extra care with these exercises if you have had hip surgery. If you experience pain in your joints or muscles while exercising, stop – check your position and try again. If the pain persists, seek medical advice. Remember: where there is pain and strain there is *no* gain.

Wheelchair

Just because some of you may have restricted movement and have to sit down for long periods or are in a wheelchair, it doesn't mean exercise is out of the question. Even simple exercise has many positive benefits for everyday life like strengthening your body and alleviating the pain of arthritis, and with the release of endorphins when you exercise it can make you feel happier.

But for your own safety, please ensure the breaks of your wheelchair are on, sit upright and if required strap up. If you do have feeling in your lower limbs place your feet comfortably on the floor. For those of you more mobile, please place your upright chair against a wall for support for these exercises.

72. CHAIR MARCH

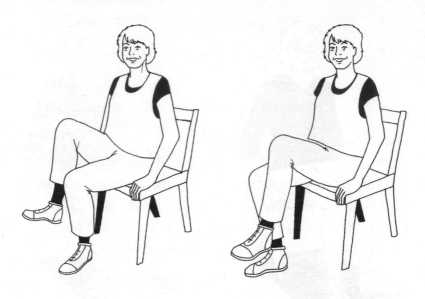

To warm up and prepare for exercise: sit tall holding the sides of a sturdy upright, armless chair. Lift your right foot up as high as possible and place it down again with control. Lift your left foot up and back down. Continue lifting each foot alternately and placing them down with control. Build to a rhythm that is comfortable for you. Continue for 30 seconds.

73. ANKLE FLIP FLAP

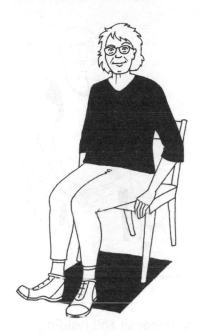 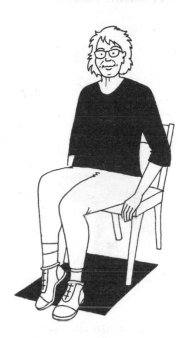

To mobilise ankles and feet: sit tall away from the back of the chair and hold on to the sides. Place the heel of your right foot on the floor, then lift the heel up and put your toes down on the same spot. Repeat this flip flap movement five times with each leg.

74. ARM SWINGS

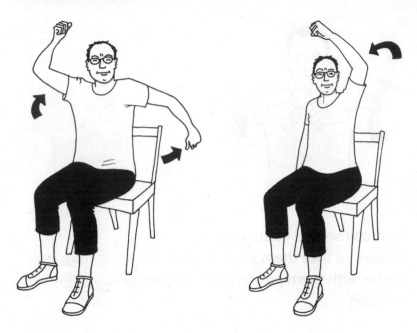

To warm up and mobilise your upper body: sit tall, away from the chair back. Place your feet flat on the floor below your knees, hip-width apart. Bend your elbows and swing your arms backwards and forwards from the shoulder. Continue rhythmically twenty times.

75. ELBOW CIRCLES

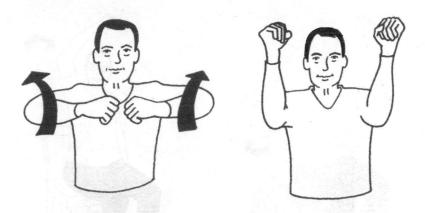

To mobilise and release tension: standing lift your elbows up take them out to your sides and simply draw circles with them pulling your shoulders back as far as possible.

76. SPINE TWISTS

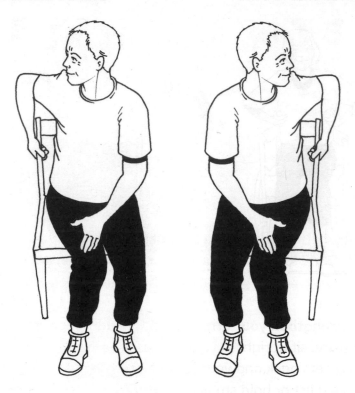

To keep your upper body supple: sit tall with your feet flat on the floor, hip-width apart. Place your left hand on your right knee and your right hand behind you on the chair back or seat. With control, turn your upper body and head to look over to your left side and hold for five seconds. Turn your upper body and head back to the centre. Repeat the exercise, placing your right hand on your left knee and looking over to your right. Hold for five seconds. Repeat on alternate sides, five times.

77. FLY LIKE A BIRD

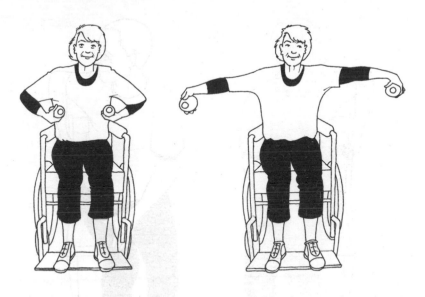

To strengthen your arms, shoulders and improve posture: sit upright in your armless chair; pull your shoulders back and your tummy in. With palms up, make a fist or hold small filled water bottles or weights. Bend your elbows, curl your arms and place your fists in front of your armpits at chest level. Now straighten your arms out wide up to shoulder level, then back in towards your chest with a controlled movement. Repeat this flying action ten times.

78. SEATED BACK STRETCH

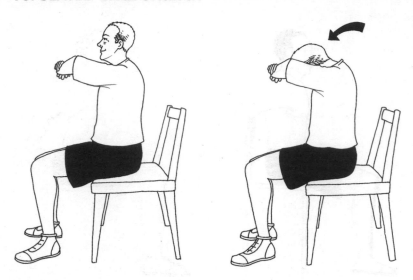

To stretch out and release tension in your back: sit in your chair. Clasp your hands around your wrists and hold them up in front of your chest. Drop your head forwards with your chin towards your chest. Lift your elbows up and out, rounding your upper back (as though you were giving someone an imaginary hug) and hold for ten seconds.

79. SEATED CHEST STRETCH

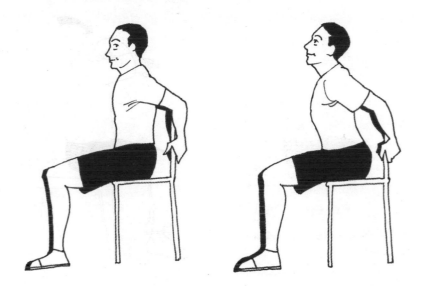

To stretch out your chest and improve your posture:
shuffle forward on your chair, hold onto the back
of chair, bring your shoulders together and stretch
out chest

80. BACK THIGH STRETCH

To stretch out back of thigh muscles: move your bottom to the front of the chair (take extra care if you have had hip surgery). Place your right foot flat on the floor then straighten your left leg out in front with your heel on the floor. Place both hands on your right thigh and sit up tall. Now lean your upper body forwards and upwards until you feel the stretch in the back of your left thigh. Hold for ten seconds. Repeat with your other leg, again holding for ten seconds.

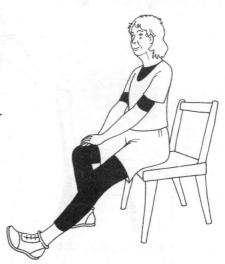

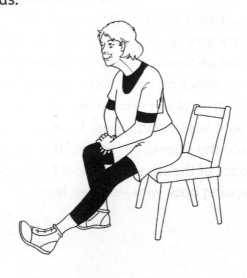

81. CALF STRETCH 1

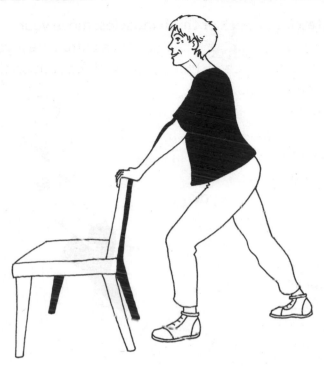

To stretch out your calf muscles (back of the lower leg): if you are able to, stand behind your sturdy upright chair and hold on firmly for support. Step back with your right leg, checking that the toes of both feet are pointing forwards. Now relax (bend) your left knee but keep your right leg straight. Press the heel of your right foot back into the floor until you feel the stretch in your right calf (back of the lower leg). Hold for ten seconds. Repeat, stepping back with your left leg.

Part 10: Stretching

Exercising our bodies is important, but so too is taking time out to stretch our muscles. Strong flexible muscles enable us to perform everyday tasks, like reaching up to high shelves, bending down to put shoes on, or twisting round to pull up zips and fasten seat belts. Flexibility and suppleness help maintain mobility into older age. Muscles should be warm in order to stretch safely, so do the following stretches after a walk, gardening, a workout or a hot bath. When you begin, take care not to overstretch, listen to your body and do what is comfortable for you. Hold the stretches – as still as you can – for five seconds, gradually increasing to 10 seconds as you progress. Hold the positions, but do not bounce.

82. CALF STRETCH 2

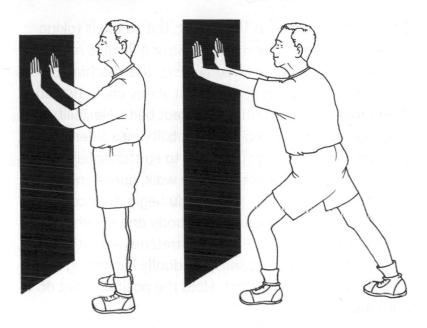

To stretch your calf muscles (back of lower leg): stand facing a wall with your feet hip-width apart. With your arms outstretched place your hands up on the wall at shoulder level. Keeping both feet facing forwards, take your right foot back and place it behind you with toes forwards. Bend your left knee. Straighten your right leg and press the heel down, and at the same time push hard against the wall with your hands. Feel the stretch in your right calf and hold steady for ten seconds. Bring your feet back together. Now, bending your right knee, take your left leg back and with your leg straight, push the left heel down to stretch your left calf. Hold for ten seconds.

83. HAMSTRING STRETCH 2

To stretch out hamstring muscles (back of thigh and bottom): stand with your feet facing forwards as before, but further back from the wall. Using the wall for support move your right foot forwards. With your knee straight, place your right heel down and pull your toes upwards. Bend your left knee, push against the wall and lift up the right side of your bottom. (If possible pull your toes upwards more to improve the stretch.) Feel the stretch in the back of your thigh and the right side of your buttocks and hold for ten seconds. Now take your left foot forwards, straighten your leg, heel down, toes up. Bend your right knee, push hard against the wall and repeat the action, stretching out the back of your left thigh and bottom. Hold for ten seconds.

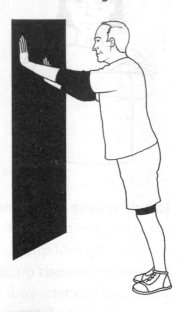

The following two stretches can be adapted for those people exercising in chairs.

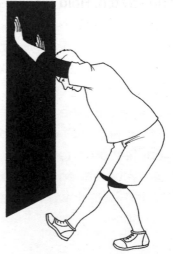

84. STANDING BACK STRETCH

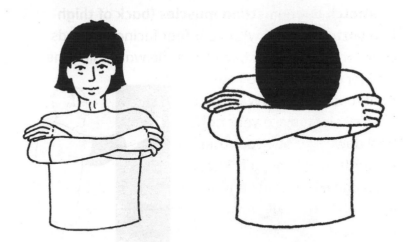

To help relieve aches and pains in the back: bend your elbows and bring your arms and hands up to shoulder level. Place your hands on your elbows and simply drop your head forwards on to your arms. Consciously round out your shoulders, your back and your neck, and enjoy the stretch. Hold for ten seconds.

85. STANDING CHEST STRETCH 2

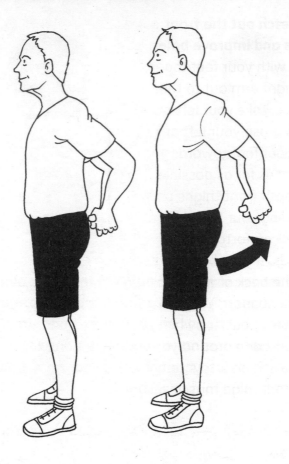

Sit or stand to stretch out your chest: take both arms behind you, grasp your hands together on your bottom and pull back your shoulders. Keep upright – try not to poke your head forwards. Now raise your hands up, bring your elbows and shoulder blades together as far as is comfortable, ensuring you lift up your rib cage. Feel the stretch across your chest and hold for ten seconds.

86. QUADS STRETCH 2

To stretch out the front of your thighs and improve balance: stand with your feet together and your right arm out to the side for balance. Take your left arm behind you to grasp your left ankle, and ease your foot towards your bottom as far as possible. Try to keep both front thighs parallel, but only bring your knees together if it feels comfortable. Hold for ten seconds. If your balance is poor, hold the back of a chair or the wall for support. You can make this stretch easier by hooking an exercise band around your foot and pulling on it to stretch out your front thigh muscles.

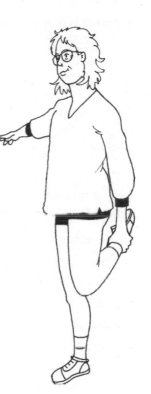

87. SIDE REACH

To stretch out the sides of your body: stand with your feet wide apart. Place your right hand on your right thigh. Bend your right knee, and with your left arm reach up and over your head as high as possible. Hold for ten seconds and feel the stretch in your left side. Repeat with the right side. You can do this exercise from a seated position by holding on to the chair seat with your right hand as you stretch up your left hand. Repeat, holding on with your left hand as you stretch up with your right.

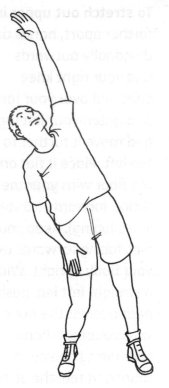

88. ADDUCTOR STRETCH (INNER THIGH MUSCLES)

To stretch out upper inside leg muscles: stand with feet further apart, hands on hips with your right foot facing diagonally outwards and your right knee bent and over your toes. Straighten your left leg and move it further to the left. Place it flat on the floor with your toes facing forwards (to stop you slipping). Keep your hips facing forwards and your body upright. With a straight left leg, push hard against the floor with your foot. Bend your right knee even 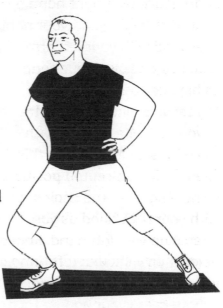 more and feel the stretch in your left inner thigh. Hold for ten seconds. Repeat on the other side with your left foot diagonally placed facing outwards and your right foot facing forwards. Hold for ten seconds.

89. ABDOMINAL STRETCH

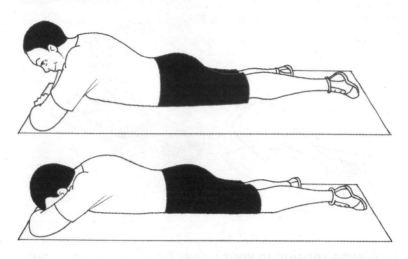

To stretch out tummy muscles and hips: lie down on your stomach. With your elbows flat on the floor in front of your shoulders, place your arms flat on the floor facing each other, one hand on top of the other. Rest your head on your hands. Take a deep breath in and, as you breathe out, lift your chest and shoulders (in a straight line) up from the floor as far as is comfortable and hold for five seconds. Keep your hips in contact with the floor at all times. You may find this stretch difficult at first, but when you are comfortable with it repeat and hold for ten seconds.

> **Warning: If you suffer from a bad back or have osteoporosis do not attempt this stretch. Caution should be taken if you have had knee or hip surgery.**

90. SHOULDER STRETCH

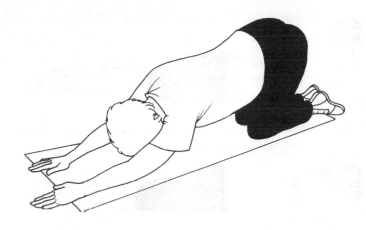

To release tension in your upper back and stretch out your shoulders: if it's comfortable, kneel on the mat, knees hip-width apart and stick your bottom up in the air. Straighten your arms and stretch them out in front of you, drop your head and carefully slide your hands forwards along the mat, lowering your chest down as far as is comfortable. Feel the stretch across your shoulders and upper back. Hold for ten seconds. Relax back on to the mat.

Warning: If you suffer from a bad back or have osteoporosis do not attempt this stretch. Caution should be taken if you have had knee or hip surgery.

91. ACTION CAT

To stretch out your spine and relieve backache: kneel comfortably on the floor, hands shoulder-width apart. Drop your head down and lifting your right knee bring it up to touch your forehead or as far as comfortable. Pull in your tummy muscles and arch up your back. Hold for 5 secs feeling the stretch across your back and shoulders. Relax and repeat with your left knee 5 times.

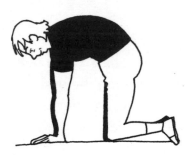 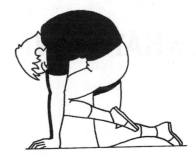

3

WHAT NOW?

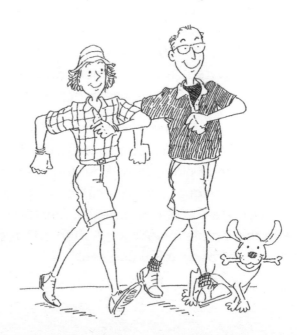

Well done; you've realised you need to make some changes, you've bought the book, read it, started to think about your new regime of healthy eating and more exercise. Well, the good news keeps getting better because now it's time to relax. Once you are calm, you can read the reminders I've included in this chapter so that it's all clear in your mind. You can then check out the list of exercises, plan which ones will be good for you, and it'll be time to sod sitting and get moving.

Relaxation exercises

Relaxation is an important part of any exercise session and it can be beneficial on its own. It's a time to wind down and chill out. Being active and exercising is all important, but our muscles and bones need time to rest and recover. Many of us continue to live fast and furious lives well into our 70s and 80s. But make no mistake, stress can be ageing. Clenched muscles restrict circulation, inhibit breathing and suppress the body's immune system, making it more vulnerable to disease. Plus, a stressed face makes us appear older.

However, you can fight off stress and relax your whole body and mind by finding space whenever possible to dedicate to quiet time. What follows is a series of simple techniques that you can practise after a walk, an exercise session or any time you feel the need, starting with this simple meditation I often do to relax and refresh my body, mind and soul.

92. VISUALISATION

Wear something loose, comfortable and warm. You can either lie on your back or sit comfortably upright in your chair. First relax with your feet flat on the floor. Rest your hands lightly on your thighs, thumbs lightly touching your second fingers, and close your eyes. Start by breathing in through the nose deep into the abdomen, and slowly out through the mouth at first, to the count of two, building to four. As you continue deep breathing take yourself off to somewhere soothing and special in your mind.

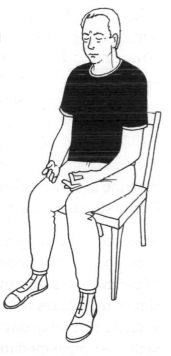

The Caribbean island of St Lucia is my vision, with cobalt blue sea and waves crashing on to rocks then rolling rhythmically up on to the beach as I breathe in time. Let yourself see, hear and feel the soft breeze, the warmth of the sun of your special place. Stay tranquil in your space for at least 10 minutes, or longer if you have the time. Finally, when you must, come to very slowly, gently shake out your limbs, open your eyes, yawn, take a couple of deep breaths and ease yourself back into your day – refreshed.

93. SIMPLY RELAX

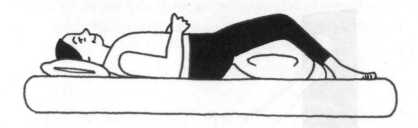

Lie back on the bed with your head supported by one or more pillows, as necessary, to improve comfort. Bend your legs a little and place another pillow behind your knees and thighs to relieve discomfort. Place your hands on your tummy with your fingertips just touching. Breathe deeply into your abdomen and out again, feeling your tummy rise and fall with your fingers. Close your eyes continue deep breathing – and relax for as long as possible.

94. ELEVATE

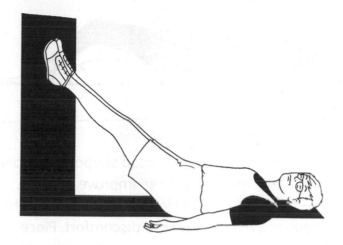

If you can't spare much time but need a quick pick-me-up, simply relieve heavy aching legs and varicose veins by encouraging the blood to flow away from the feet and legs. Whenever possible take the opportunity to elevate and rest your legs. Lie comfortably on the bed, settee or floor with a small pillow to support your head. Stretch out your legs and place them up higher on some pillows or cushions, or even the wall. Make sure your feet are higher than your heart. Do some deep breathing, in through your nose and out through your mouth, and relax for as long as you can. Your legs will thank you for some time off.

> **Warning: Do not attempt the following two positions if you have problems with knees, hips or ankles.**

95. SIT BACK

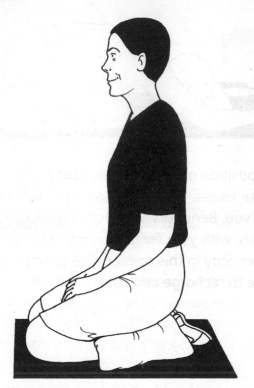

Kneel on the floor and place a cushion behind your knees. If it's possible, sit back on to it; your leg joints will be supported by the cushion. This is a comfortable position to relax in, and also one to adopt if you are gardening or working on the floor. It will ensure your joints are protected all the time.

96. WIND DOWN

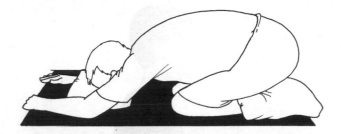

From the position above, sit back, keeping the cushion behind your knees. Place a second cushion on the floor in front of you. Bend forwards from the waist to rest on your elbows, with your forearms and head resting on the cushion. Stay in this comfortable position for as long as possible to recharge and relax.

97. WHOLE BODY STRETCH AND RELAX

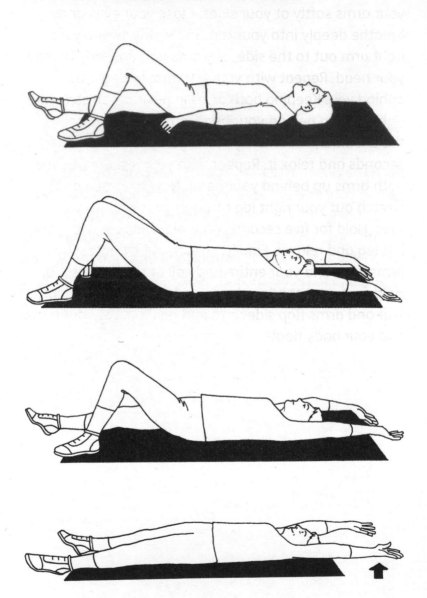

Lie back on a mat with your legs slightly apart and your arms softly at your sides. Close your eyes and breathe deeply into your tummy. Slowly sweep your right arm out to the side, onwards and upwards behind your head. Repeat with your left arm, taking it up behind you. Keeping both arms in position, stretch your right arm up behind your head, stretching through the shoulder, chest and your fingertips. Hold for five seconds and relax it. Repeat with your left arm. Leave both arms up behind your head. Now lengthen and stretch out your right leg through your knee to your toes. Hold for five seconds and relax. Repeat with your left leg and relax it. Finally, stretch out through your arms, legs and your entire body all at the same time. Hold for five seconds, release and relax. Let your legs, feet and arms flop sideways and go limp. Let your mind and your body float!

Your daily vitality programme

The world we live in is one in which:

- Inactivity is a major cause of the changes that everyone, many doctors included, believe are caused by ageing.

- By becoming more active people can increase their vitality and regain the level of fitness they had 10 years earlier.

- This can happen in your 60s, 70s, 80s and probably your 90s too. It applies to all four aspects of physical fitness – strength, stamina, suppleness and skill – and increased levels of activity have many psychological benefits too.

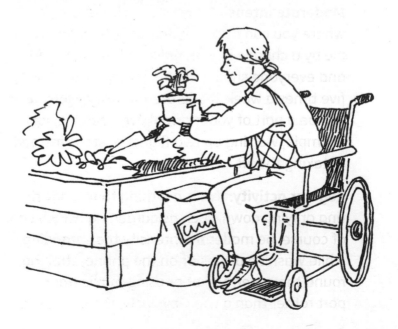

There are four levels of activity, all of them beneficial. They are classified as follows:

- **High intensity:** you can do nothing but flop on the ground after high-intensity activity. Fitness experts say that even 30 seconds of high-intensity exercise is beneficial. It is usually recommended for younger people and probably best avoided by people over 60.

- **Vigorous intensity:** activities such as fast swimming or cycling up a steep hill will leave you too breathless to speak normally, but not in a state of collapse. This level of activity is good for people over 60 and you should aim to do something like this at least twice a week.

- **Moderate intensity:** this is exercise at a level where you can definitely feel its effect, for example by a change in your pulse or breathing rate, and everyone should aim for this level of activity five times a week. Moderate-intensity exercise can be a part of your normal everyday life; for example, walking up two flights of stairs instead of taking the lift.

- **Regular activity:** this is anything that is not sitting or lying down, such as gardening (which can, of course, be moderate intensity too), standing while washing dishes or on the phone, strolling round the supermarket or using public transport rather than a car. Obviously, the amount of energy used in regular everyday activity is not as great as in moderate-intensity activities, but because you can do it for so long it is very beneficial, particularly for controlling your weight.

Here is a summary of what is needed in terms of activity each week:

Level of activity	Frequency
Vigorous intensity	At least twice a week
Moderate intensity	At least five times a week
Regular activity	Try to build an extra hour of standing and moving every day

As you have read as far as this, it seems likely you are serious about your health. Great: it's time to commit! Before you start to plan your campaign, it is important to remember that different types of activity help develop the four S's: strength, stamina, suppleness and skill. Don't just do a bit more than you currently do, get obsessional about it: get walking, more and briskly; commit to your daily vitality; get up, if and whenever you can; get lively, go back to sports and active hobbies, or take up new ones.

GET OBSESSIONAL

The scientific evidence about the benefits of training is very strong, and has been for decades. Professor Roy J. Shephard, author of *Ageing, Physical Activity and*

Health, uses the word 'training' frequently, and many of the research projects he quotes are characterised by the type of regular activity designed to increase strength, stamina, suppleness and skill in just the way that people train for competitive sport. Examples of the types of exercise that research subjects in their 60s, 70s, 80s and 90s did are:

- One supervised and two unsupervised sessions of 'weight-bearing' physical activity per week

- A circuit of 12 resistance exercises three times per week for 50 weeks

This type of structured exercise programme can rightly be called training, but don't be put off by the name; we are training not for competitive sport but for a better quality of life both now and in the decades to come:

- People in their 60s need to train for better quality of life in their 60s, 70s, 80s and 90s

- People in their 70s need to train for better quality of life in their 70s, 80s and 90s

- People in their 80s need to train for better quality of life in their 80s and 90s

- People in their 90s need to train for better quality of life in their 90s, and if you are fit in your 90s you will carry this forwards into LATT – 'Life after the telegram'!

Sportsmen and women are obsessional about training – Daley Thompson said that he always trained on Christmas Day, because he knew his competitors would be having a day off – and if you are training for your 60s, 70s, 80s, 90s, and beyond, you need to get obsessional about standing and walking.

YOUR FUTURE

Well done if you are embarking on your new exercise programme, possibly for the first time in years. Exercise should be comfortable and fun, so why not also consider joining a fitness class for older people? Most sports centres have qualified instructors who specialise in classes for the over-60s and those less mobile. You could try a t'ai chi or Pilates or Alexander technique class, or perhaps think about suggesting or introducing an exercise class to any club you might already belong to.

As the popular saying goes, 'use it or lose it', and it applies to both body and mind. I'm a firm believer in exercising the mind as well as the body in order to function efficiently. Being active can transform your lifestyle .... so down with sofas and up with stairs! Remember, age is mind over matter ... and if you don't mind it doesn't matter. Be happy and be healthy, whatever your age.

YOUR ESSENTIAL 5-A-DAY EXERCISE PLAN

If you haven't exercised for a while or have physical limitations, why not make a simple and personal 5-a-day exercise plan to motivate you? Here are a few suggestions. When you feel comfortable doing the exercises you could look through the sections in the book applicable to your needs, add others and increase your plan to a 10-a-day exercise regime!

BEGINNERS
- Wake up monkey stretch (page 55)
- Side reach and stretch (page 62)
- Arms back (page 66)
- High lifts (page 87)
- Tummy tuck (page 91)

MOBILITY PROBLEMS
- Wake up monkey stretch (page 55)
- Shoulder circles (page 61)

- Lift and stretch 1 (page 65)
- Lift off (page 82)
- Shoulder stretch (page 157)

POSTURE

- Wake up monkey stretch (page 55)
- Flings (page 75)
- Ballet (page 84)
- V for victory (page 132)
- Wall press-ups (page 123)

STRENGTH

- Wake up monkey stretch (page 55)
- Biceps three of a kind (page 72)
- The flyer (page 68)
- Bottom lift (page 89)
- Row the boat (page 134)

FLEXIBILITY

- Wake up monkey strength (page 55)
- Quads stretch 1 (page 104)
- Pull-aways (page 110)
- Side reach (page 154)
- Action cat (page 158)

List of exercises

Part 10: Stretching

Relaxation exercises

ABOUT THE AUTHORS

Diana Moran. Famous for being the BBC's Green Goddess fitness expert in the 80s, Diana Moran still works as a health and fitness guru, broadcaster, and writer. In her late 70s Diana practices, what she preaches – remaining fit and healthy by staying active year to year.

Diana has published 11 health-related books and has many videos and DVDs to her credit. She continues to educate women of all ages on keeping healthy, but especially targets her message to 'Women Who Weren't Born Yesterday'. She says, 'Women like me have so much to do in the rest of our lives – we're not as young as we used to be, but we're not as old as some people think we should be! We know that staying healthy means we enjoy our lives so much more – and there are no quick fixes – we weren't born yesterday!'

Unbelievably, 2017 will see Diana enjoying her 78th birthday – despite looking at least thirty years younger! She is a testimony to healthy living and has been dubbed Britain's Jane Fonda!

Sir Muir Gray has worked in public heath for over 40 years. The first phase of his career focused on disease prevention, particularly helping people stop smoking and population ageing.

He later went on to develop screening programmes in the NHS for pregnant women, children and older people. This included offering men aged sixty-five screening for abdominal aortic aneurysm and, for both men and women, colorectal cancer.

Muir also developed services to bring knowledge to patients and professionals via NHS choices. During this period he was appointed Chief Knowledge Officer of the NHS and was awarded both a CBE and later a Knighthood for services for the NHS.

ACKNOWLEDGEMENTS

Diana Moran

My thanks go to my erstwhile friend and agent Tony Fitzpatrick, who has introduced me to the wonderful team at Bloomsbury and the wisdom and understanding from my editors Charlotte Croft and Sarah Skipper. Their belief in supporting the over 70s has been inspirational and a gift to the next generations ahead. As the wise Gautama Buddha is credited as saying, 'To keep the body in good health is a duty – otherwise we shall not be able to keep our minds strong and clear...' I wish all my readers the wisdom to live a healthy old age.

Muir Gray

I would like to thank Rosemary Lees who is, like me, in the prime of life and who typed as well as ever converting my scrawl to readable text. The team at Bloomsbury has managed the project very well and Tony Fitzpatrick has edited the two authors' work so that it flows seamlessly.

INDEX

Page numbers in *italics* refer to figures